# STORIES FROM THE NICU

## VOLUME 3

## DR. ERIN SMITH

FREE REIGN
Publishing

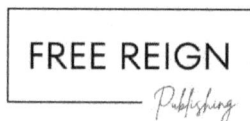

FREE REIGN
Publishing

# CONTENTS

# INTRODUCTION

In the dimly lit corridors of the Neonatal Intensive Care Unit (NICU), life is a delicate balance between hope and uncertainty. Every breath, every heartbeat, and every tiny cry holds profound significance. Here, in this unique space, the smallest and most vulnerable members of our society begin their fight for life, surrounded by an army of dedicated healthcare professionals who strive to give them a fighting chance.

Each story is a testament to the resilience of the human spirit and the power of love, science, and unwavering dedication. *Stories From the NICU* is a collection of experiences I've gathered over the years from fellow doctors and nurses, offering a window into the world where the fragility of life is met with extraordinary strength and compassion.

This book is not just a series of medical cases; it is a chronicle of the human journey at its most raw and vulnerable. Through these narratives, you will meet families whose lives have been forever changed by their time in the NICU. You will encounter the triumphs and challenges faced by the tiny warriors who have overcome insurmountable odds. And you will gain insight into the tireless efforts of the medical staff who work around the clock, driven by a deep sense of duty and compassion.

Each chapter in this book is a story of hope, resilience, and the indomitable spirit of both the infants and their families. From the first moments of life, filled with uncertainty, to the joyous milestones that mark their journey home, these tales will touch your heart and inspire your soul.

*Stories From the NICU* is a tribute to the strength of the human spirit and a celebration of the incredible advances in neonatal medicine. It is my hope that through these stories, you will gain a deeper appreciation for the miracles that happen every day in the NICU and the unwavering commitment of those who dedicate their lives to saving the tiniest of patients.

Welcome to the world of the NICU and pediatric medicine, where every life is a story worth telling.

With heartfelt gratitude and respect,

Dr. Erin Smith

# CHAPTER ONE

## NEONATAL LUPUS

I REMEMBER THE PATIENT WELL. It was a challenging case that tested all my skills as a NICU doctor. The patient, a newborn, presented with symptoms that initially seemed typical for our ward but quickly evolved into something far more complex.

The patient was born at 38 weeks gestation to a mother with a known history of autoimmune disease. This immediately raised red flags, and we prepared for possible complications. At birth, the patient appeared relatively healthy, with Apgar scores of 8 and 9 at one and five minutes, respectively. However, within a few hours, the patient began to exhibit signs of distress.

The first indication of trouble was a rash. The patient developed erythematous lesions on the face and scalp, which spread to the trunk and limbs. These lesions had a characteristic appearance, suggestive of a butterfly rash across the cheeks, which immediately made me suspect neonatal lupus erythematosus (NLE). I ordered a full workup to confirm the diagnosis and rule out other potential causes.

The laboratory tests were telling. The patient tested positive for anti-Ro (SSA) and anti-La (SSB) antibodies. These antibodies, transferred from the mother, confirmed the diagnosis of neonatal lupus. The patient also exhibited signs of thrombocytopenia, with platelet counts significantly below normal levels, and mild anemia. Given the combination of clinical presentation and lab results, the diagnosis of neonatal lupus erythematosus was unequivocal.

Neonatal lupus is a rare condition, and it was imperative to monitor the patient closely for any potential complications, particularly those affecting the heart. Approximately 15-30% of infants with neonatal lupus develop congenital heart block (CHB), a serious condition that can be life-threatening. An immediate echocardiogram was ordered to assess cardiac function. The echocardiogram revealed a first-degree heart block, which, although concerning, was not as severe as a complete block.

The treatment plan was multi-faceted, aiming to manage the symptoms and prevent further complications. The patient's skin lesions were treated with a topical corticosteroid to reduce inflammation. For the thrombocytopenia, intravenous immunoglobulin (IVIG) was administered to boost platelet counts. The anemia was mild and did not require immediate intervention, but we planned to monitor hemoglobin levels closely.

Given the heart block, we needed to be vigilant. Although the patient only had a first-degree block, the risk of progression to a more severe block was present. We decided on a conservative approach with close monitoring, including frequent electrocardiograms (ECGs) and echocardiograms. If the block progressed, we were prepared to initiate corticosteroid therapy or, in the worst-case scenario, consider a pacemaker.

In addition to these treatments, the patient received supportive care, including phototherapy for mild jaundice, which is common in newborns but can be exacerbated by hemolysis in conditions like neonatal lupus. We also provided nutritional support through a nasogastric tube, as the patient had difficulty feeding due to fatigue and poor suckling reflexes.

Throughout the treatment, the patient's condition remained stable but required constant vigilance. The skin lesions gradually improved with the corticosteroid treatment, and platelet counts increased following the IVIG administration. However, the heart block remained a concern. We conducted daily ECGs and weekly echocardiograms to monitor any changes.

After a week in the NICU, the patient showed signs of improvement. The platelet count stabilized within the normal range, and the hemoglobin levels, while still low, were gradually improving. The skin lesions were healing, leaving only slight discoloration. However, the first-degree heart block persisted.

Given the patient's stable condition, we began to transition from intensive monitoring to a more regular care routine. The patient continued to receive topical corticosteroids for the skin and was maintained on a watchful waiting protocol for the heart block. We educated the parents extensively about the signs of worsening heart block and the importance of regular follow-up with a pediatric cardiologist.

Despite the challenges, the patient's progress was encouraging. The immune-mediated complications of neonatal lupus were managed effectively with the treatments provided, and no new symptoms emerged. The patient remained in the NICU for three weeks, during which we observed steady improvement in all parameters.

On the day of discharge from the NICU, the patient's skin lesions had almost completely resolved, with just a few residual marks that were expected to fade over time. The platelet count and hemoglobin levels were within acceptable ranges, and the patient was feeding well, demonstrating adequate weight gain.

The first-degree heart block persisted, but there were no signs of progression. The patient was discharged with a detailed care plan that included regular follow-ups with a pediatrician and a pediatric cardiologist. The parents were instructed to monitor the patient closely for any signs of cardiac distress and were provided with information on the potential long-term implications of neonatal lupus.

In the NICU, we did our best to provide comprehensive care and support. The patient's case was a reminder of the complexities and challenges of neonatal medicine. While the immediate crisis was managed, the long-term outcome would depend on careful monitoring and follow-up care. The patient left the NICU stable and with a good prognosis, but the journey was far from over.

# CHAPTER TWO

### ANEMIA

IT WAS an ordinary day in the NICU, or as ordinary as a day can be in a place where every moment teeters between life and death. I was going through my routine checks when the next patient arrived. The patient, a newborn, had been transferred to our hospital for further evaluation and treatment due to suspected severe anemia.

Upon initial observation, the patient appeared unusually pale and lethargic, a stark contrast to the more vigorous infants typically seen. This presentation, combined with a significantly elevated heart rate, indicated the urgency of the situation. We proceeded with a complete blood count (CBC) to quantify the extent of the anemia. The results were alarming. The patient's hemoglobin level was markedly low at 6 g/dL, with a hematocrit level of 18%. The normal range for a newborn is between 14 to 20 g/dL for hemoglobin and 42% to 65% for hematocrit. Clearly, the patient was in critical condition.

Further blood tests were conducted to determine the cause of the anemia. A reticulocyte count revealed a lower than expected number of reticulocytes, suggesting that the anemia was due to a production problem rather than a hemolytic process or blood loss. Serum ferritin, iron, and total iron-binding capacity (TIBC) tests were ordered to evaluate iron levels. The results showed severely depleted iron stores, pointing to iron deficiency as the underlying cause of the anemia.

With the diagnosis confirmed, our immediate focus was to stabilize the patient. The first step was to administer a blood transfusion to quickly raise the hemoglobin level and alleviate the symptoms of anemia. We transfused 10 mL/kg of packed red blood cells (PRBCs) over three hours, closely monitoring the patient for any signs of transfusion reactions, such as fever, rash, or respiratory distress. Thankfully, the transfusion proceeded without complications, and the patient's hemoglobin level rose to a more stable 10 g/dL.

While the transfusion provided temporary relief, it was essential to address the root cause of the anemia to ensure long-term recovery. Given the iron deficiency indicated by the lab results, an iron supplementation regimen was initiated. We prescribed oral ferrous sulfate at a dose of 3 mg/kg/day, divided into three doses. This approach would help replenish the iron stores and support the production of new red blood cells.

We also arranged for parenteral nutrition (PN) because the patient was too weak to feed adequately by mouth. The PN included iron dextran, a more direct form of iron supplementation that bypasses the gastrointestinal tract. This method ensured that the patient received the necessary nutrients without further taxing their compromised digestive system.

In addition to iron supplementation, we monitored the patient for any potential complications arising from severe anemia and its treatment. Regular CBCs were performed to track the patient's response to the interventions. We also kept a close watch on vital signs, including heart rate, respiratory rate, and oxygen saturation, to detect any early signs of deterioration.

Over the next few days, the patient showed gradual improvement. The pallor began to fade, and there was a noticeable increase in activity levels. Follow-up blood tests indicated a slow but steady rise in hemoglobin and hematocrit levels, confirming the effectiveness of the treatment plan. The reticulocyte count also increased, indicating that the patient's bone marrow was responding well and beginning to produce new red blood cells.

Despite these positive signs, the patient remained in a vulnerable state. It was crucial to prevent any infections, as the immune system was still compromised due to the anemia. We maintained strict aseptic techniques and limited the number of visitors to reduce the risk of exposure to pathogens.

A key aspect of the patient's care involved regular multidisciplinary team meetings. These included neonatologists, hematologists, dietitians, and nurses to ensure a comprehensive approach to treatment. Each member contributed their expertise to fine-tune the care plan and address any emerging issues promptly.

As days turned into weeks, the patient's condition continued to stabilize. The iron supplementation regimen was gradually adjusted based on the patient's progress and blood test results. We also started to introduce small amounts of fortified formula feeds to transition from parenteral to enteral nutrition. This step was critical for long-term growth and development, as it helped the patient's digestive system adapt and function properly.

Throughout this period, we remained vigilant for any signs of relapse or complications. Regular follow-up appointments were scheduled to monitor the patient's progress and make necessary adjustments to the treatment plan. Education for the family was also a priority, ensuring they understood the importance of adherence to the iron supplementation regimen and the need for ongoing medical supervision.

By the end of the patient's stay in the NICU, the hemoglobin and hematocrit levels were within the normal range for a newborn. The reticulocyte count was also within normal limits, indicating a healthy bone marrow response. The patient was more active and feeding well, with no signs of respiratory distress or other complications.

The day finally arrived when we could discharge the patient from the NICU. Although the patient still required close follow-up and continued iron supplementation, the immediate crisis had been resolved. The patient's parents were given detailed instructions on medication administration, signs of potential relapse, and the importance of regular pediatric visits.

While the journey was far from over, the progress made during the NICU stay laid a strong foundation for future health and development.

As a NICU doctor, these experiences are both challenging and rewarding, constantly reinforcing the critical nature of our work in giving these fragile lives a fighting chance.

# CHAPTER THREE

## BRONCHOPULMONARY DYSPLASIA

AS A NEONATOLOGIST IN THE NICU, I encountered many challenging cases, but few were as intricate and demanding as that of the patient with Bronchopulmonary Dysplasia (BPD). The patient was born at 26 weeks gestation, a premature infant weighing just under 1,000 grams. Immediately after birth, the patient required intubation and mechanical ventilation due to respiratory distress syndrome, a common condition in preterm infants due to insufficient surfactant production in the lungs.

In the first days of life, the patient's condition was closely monitored. Despite initial stabilization with surfactant replacement therapy and continuous positive airway pressure (CPAP), the patient continued to exhibit significant respiratory distress. The ventilator settings had to be frequently adjusted to maintain adequate oxygenation and ventilation. High-frequency oscillatory ventilation (HFOV) was employed to minimize lung injury and optimize gas exchange.

By the second week, the patient was still dependent on mechanical ventilation. Chest radiographs showed typical signs of evolving BPD: diffuse haziness, interstitial thickening, and areas of hyperinflation and atelectasis. Blood gases often showed mixed respiratory and metabolic acidosis, indicative of ongoing respiratory compromise and the patient's struggle to adapt.

To manage BPD, we initiated a multi-faceted treatment plan. The cornerstone of the treatment was the gradual weaning from mechanical ventilation to non-invasive respiratory support. This process was slow and required meticulous adjustments to avoid both hypoxia and hyperoxia, which could further damage the delicate lung tissue.

Corticosteroids were considered early in the course but were deferred until the fourth week of life due to potential adverse effects on neurodevelopment. When initiated, a low-dose dexamethasone regimen was used to facilitate extubation. The patient responded with some improvement in lung function, and we were able to transition from HFOV to conventional ventilation, and eventually to nasal CPAP.

Nutrition was another critical aspect of the treatment. To support lung growth and repair, the patient received fortified human milk through a nasogastric tube. Total parenteral nutrition (TPN) was initially used to ensure adequate caloric intake, with a gradual transition to enteral feeds as the patient's gastrointestinal function matured. The diet was high in protein, calories, and essential nutrients to promote overall growth and development.

Diuretics, such as furosemide and spironolactone, were prescribed to manage fluid balance and reduce pulmonary edema, a common complication in BPD. Regular electrolyte monitoring was necessary to prevent imbalances and ensure the patient's stability. Inhaled bronchodilators, such as albuterol, were used intermittently to relieve bronchospasm and improve airflow.

The patient's condition was closely monitored through frequent arterial blood gas analyses, pulse oximetry, and capnography to ensure adequate ventilation and oxygenation. Echocardiograms were performed periodically to assess for pulmonary hypertension, a common comorbidity in BPD patients. Fortunately, the patient did not develop significant pulmonary hypertension, allowing us to focus on optimizing respiratory support and nutrition.

Despite these interventions, progress was slow. The

patient's oxygen requirements fluctuated, and we faced several episodes of respiratory exacerbations triggered by infections. Each episode required a tailored approach, including antibiotics for suspected sepsis and adjustments in respiratory support. The patient's fragile condition made them susceptible to secondary complications such as retinopathy of prematurity (ROP), which necessitated regular ophthalmologic evaluations and eventually laser therapy to prevent vision loss.

By the sixth week, the patient showed signs of gradual improvement. The corticosteroid therapy helped reduce lung inflammation, allowing us to decrease ventilator support progressively. Weaning off mechanical ventilation was a delicate balance of reducing settings while ensuring the patient could maintain adequate gas exchange. Once off the ventilator, the patient continued on nasal CPAP with supplemental oxygen.

The patient's weight gain and growth parameters were closely tracked. Nutritional support was adjusted based on weekly growth assessments and laboratory results. Multidisciplinary rounds, including respiratory therapists, nutritionists, and pharmacists, ensured a comprehensive approach to the patient's care. The collaboration was crucial for addressing the complex needs of BPD management.

Over the subsequent weeks, the patient continued to

make incremental progress. The need for diuretics decreased as the lung condition stabilized, and we began transitioning from nasal CPAP to high-flow nasal cannula (HFNC). This transition required careful titration of flow rates and $FiO_2$ to maintain adequate oxygenation while promoting the patient's own respiratory efforts.

Throughout the course of treatment, we faced numerous challenges, including managing the delicate balance of fluid intake, preventing nosocomial infections, and addressing the patient's ongoing need for respiratory support. Regular follow-ups with pulmonologists and cardiologists were scheduled to monitor for late complications of BPD, such as chronic lung disease and pulmonary hypertension.

After several months in the NICU, the patient reached a point where they could be weaned off oxygen during daytime hours, requiring it only during sleep and feedings. This was a significant milestone, indicating a marked improvement in lung function and overall stability.

Eventually, the patient was able to transition to low-flow nasal cannula oxygen therapy, and preparations for discharge began. The patient required extensive family education and training on home oxygen use, signs of respiratory distress, and the importance of follow-up appointments. Coordination with home healthcare services was essential to ensure a smooth transition from the hospital to home care.

By the time of discharge, the patient was stable on minimal respiratory support, showing steady growth and development appropriate for their corrected gestational age. While the journey with BPD was far from over, the patient had overcome the most critical period of their illness, thanks to the comprehensive and coordinated efforts of the NICU team.

The experience underscored the complexities of managing severe BPD in preterm infants and the importance of a multidisciplinary approach to address the myriad challenges these patients face.

# CHAPTER FOUR

## PERSISTENT PULMONARY HYPERTENSION OF THE NEWBORN

THE PATIENT WAS BORN at 38 weeks gestation via emergency cesarean section after a prolonged labor that showed signs of fetal distress. The Apgar scores were low at birth, indicating severe asphyxia. The baby was immediately transferred to our NICU for further evaluation and management.

Upon arrival in the NICU, the patient was noted to be in significant respiratory distress. The baby's skin had a cyanotic hue, and there was noticeable grunting, flaring of the nostrils, and retractions of the chest wall with each breath. Initial assessment revealed a heart rate of 180 beats per minute, a respiratory rate of 70 breaths per minute, and an oxygen saturation of 75% on room air. Auscultation of the chest revealed diminished breath sounds bilaterally with a pronounced cardiac murmur.

Given the patient's presentation, the immediate concern was Persistent Pulmonary Hypertension of the Newborn (PPHN). This condition occurs when the newborn's circulation system doesn't adapt to breathing outside the womb. In PPHN, the blood vessels in the lungs remain constricted, leading to poor oxygenation of the blood.

The diagnosis was further supported by a chest X-ray, which showed clear lung fields, ruling out other causes of respiratory distress such as pneumonia or meconium aspiration syndrome. An echocardiogram was performed urgently, which confirmed the presence of elevated pulmonary artery pressures and right-to-left shunting at the level of the patent ductus arteriosus and foramen ovale, hallmark signs of PPHN.

The first step in managing PPHN was to optimize oxygenation and ventilation. The patient was immediately placed on mechanical ventilation with high levels of oxygen. A blood gas analysis revealed severe hypoxemia and acidosis, which needed correction. The ventilator settings were adjusted to provide high-frequency oscillatory ventilation (HFOV) to improve oxygenation without causing lung injury. HFOV is often used in severe cases of PPHN as it helps to open the alveoli and improve gas exchange more effectively than conventional ventilation.

In addition to mechanical ventilation, the patient was started on inhaled nitric oxide (iNO) therapy. Nitric oxide is a potent vasodilator that, when inhaled, selectively dilates the pulmonary blood vessels, reducing pulmonary hypertension and improving oxygenation. The initial dose was set at 20 parts per million (ppm), with close monitoring of the patient's response.

The patient was also given a surfactant replacement therapy. Surfactant is a substance that helps keep the lungs' air sacs open and is often deficient in infants with PPHN. The administration of surfactant aimed to improve lung compliance and reduce the work of breathing.

Given the severity of the patient's condition, it was crucial to maintain adequate systemic blood pressure to ensure proper perfusion of vital organs. The patient was started on an intravenous infusion of dopamine and dobutamine, both of which are inotropic agents that support cardiac output and blood pressure. Dopamine was administered at a dose of 5 micrograms per kilogram per minute, and dobutamine was given at a dose of 10 micrograms per kilogram per minute. These medications were titrated based on continuous monitoring of the patient's blood pressure and urine output.

Fluid management was another critical aspect of care. The patient was given intravenous fluids to maintain hydration and electrolyte balance. However, fluid overload was carefully avoided to prevent exacerbation of pulmonary edema. The fluid intake was meticulously calculated, and diuretics such as furosemide were administered as needed to manage fluid status.

In addition to the primary treatments, supportive care measures were implemented. The patient was placed in a thermoneutral environment to prevent cold stress, which could worsen pulmonary hypertension. Nutritional support was provided through total parenteral nutrition (TPN) initially, and as the patient's condition stabilized, enteral feeding was gradually introduced via a nasogastric tube.

Continuous monitoring was essential in managing the patient's condition. The patient was connected to a multi-parameter monitor that tracked heart rate, respiratory rate, blood pressure, oxygen saturation, and end-tidal carbon dioxide levels. Regular blood gas analyses were performed to assess the effectiveness of the ventilation and oxygenation strategies.

Despite the aggressive treatment, the patient's condition remained critical for several days. The oxygenation index (OI), a measure of the severity of hypoxemia and the effectiveness of the treatment, fluctuated but gradually showed signs of improvement. The inhaled nitric oxide therapy was slowly weaned off over the course of a week as the patient's pulmonary pressures began to normalize, and the oxygenation improved.

As the patient's respiratory status stabilized, the ventilator settings were gradually reduced. The high-frequency oscillatory ventilation was transitioned to conventional mechanical ventilation, and then to non-invasive ventilation modes such as continuous positive airway pressure (CPAP). Eventually, the patient was able to maintain adequate oxygenation on supplemental oxygen via nasal cannula.

Throughout this period, the patient received regular echocardiograms to monitor the pulmonary artery pressures and the resolution of the right-to-left shunting. By the end of the second week, the echocardiogram showed significant improvement with near normalization of pulmonary pressures and no evidence of shunting.

Once the patient's respiratory and hemodynamic status was stable, attention was turned to feeding and growth. The patient was gradually advanced from naso-gastric tube feeds to oral feeding. Breast milk was forti-fied to ensure adequate caloric intake and support growth and development. The patient's weight gain and overall health were closely monitored.

After three weeks of intensive care and gradual weaning of supportive treatments, the patient showed remarkable improvement. The oxygen requirement decreased steadily, and the patient was eventually weaned off supplemental oxygen. The echocardiogram at discharge showed normal pulmonary pressures and no evidence of structural heart defects or persistent shunting.

The patient was discharged from the NICU at 28 days of life in stable condition. Follow-up care was arranged with a pediatric cardiologist and a pulmonologist to monitor the patient's progress and ensure no long-term sequelae of PPHN. The patient left the NICU with a good prognosis, having overcome the critical period of severe pulmonary hypertension.

The patient's successful recovery was a testament to the effectiveness of the comprehensive and aggressive treatment strategy employed in the NICU.

---

# CHAPTER FIVE

IT WAS A PARTICULARLY CHALLENGING day in the NICU, the kind of day where the air felt heavy with anticipation and anxiety. I had just finished reviewing my rounds when I was alerted to a new admission. A preterm infant, born at 28 weeks gestation, was brought into our unit with signs of severe respiratory distress. The tiny patient, swaddled in a blanket, was rushed to the intensive care incubator. The situation demanded immediate attention and a precise, methodical approach.

Upon initial examination, the infant exhibited classic symptoms of Respiratory Distress Syndrome (RDS). The telltale signs were all there: rapid, shallow breathing, grunting sounds with each exhalation, and a distinct blue tinge to the skin, indicating cyanosis. The heart rate was elevated, and the oxygen saturation levels were perilously low.

The first step was to secure the airway and ensure adequate oxygenation. We administered a fraction of inspired oxygen (FiO2) via a nasal continuous positive airway pressure (CPAP) machine. CPAP is a crucial first-line intervention in RDS as it helps keep the alveoli open, improving gas exchange and reducing the work of breathing.

While the CPAP machine delivered steady, gentle pressure to the infant's lungs, I proceeded with a more thorough diagnostic evaluation. A chest X-ray was performed to confirm the presence of RDS. The radiograph revealed a characteristic "ground glass" appearance with air bronchograms, which are hallmarks of this condition. The diagnosis was clear: the patient was suffering from hyaline membrane disease, another term for RDS, caused by the immaturity of the lungs and the lack of surfactant.

Surfactant is a substance that reduces surface tension within the alveoli, preventing them from collapsing. In preterm infants, the production of surfactant is often insufficient, leading to the development of RDS. Given the severity of the patient's condition, exogenous surfactant therapy was imperative.

With the consent of the parents obtained earlier, I

prepared for the administration of the surfactant. The drug of choice in our NICU is a natural surfactant extract, administered intratracheally. This process involves intubating the infant and delivering the surfactant directly into the lungs. Intubation in such a fragile patient is a delicate procedure, requiring precision and a steady hand. Once the endotracheal tube was correctly placed, we administered the surfactant in small, controlled aliquots, carefully monitoring the patient's response.

The immediate goal was to stabilize the patient and improve oxygenation. Following the surfactant administration, we adjusted the ventilator settings to optimize the patient's breathing. The initial response was promising: the oxygen saturation levels began to rise, and the grunting diminished. However, this was just the beginning of a long and arduous journey.

The treatment plan for the patient was multifaceted, addressing both the immediate respiratory needs and the overall well-being of the infant. In addition to the respiratory support, we initiated a regimen of intravenous fluids to maintain hydration and electrolyte balance. Preterm infants have underdeveloped renal function and are at risk of fluid imbalances, so meticulous monitoring of fluid intake and output was essential.

We also started a course of antibiotics. Preterm

infants are particularly vulnerable to infections due to their immature immune systems. Prophylactic antibiotics are often administered to prevent or treat potential sepsis, a common and life-threatening complication in the NICU.

Nutritional support was another critical aspect of the patient's care. Enteral feeding, using a nasogastric tube, was initiated to provide the necessary calories and nutrients for growth and development. Human milk fortifier was added to the breast milk to increase the caloric density, ensuring the patient received adequate nutrition despite the challenges of preterm feeding.

Monitoring was continuous and intensive. The patient's vital signs, blood gases, and laboratory parameters were closely observed to detect any signs of deterioration or complications. The arterial blood gases showed gradual improvement, indicating better oxygenation and ventilation. The X-rays taken at intervals showed a slow but steady clearing of the lungs, a positive sign that the surfactant was working and the lungs were beginning to function more effectively.

Despite these improvements, the patient's condition remained precarious. Preterm infants with RDS are at high risk for several complications, including bronchopulmonary dysplasia (BPD), patent ductus arteriosus (PDA), and intraventricular hemorrhage (IVH). We conducted regular cranial ultrasounds to monitor for any signs of IVH, a common and serious complication in very low birth weight infants. Fortunately, the ultrasounds showed no evidence of bleeding.

The patient also underwent regular echocardiograms to check for PDA, a condition where the ductus arteriosus, a blood vessel in the heart that is supposed to close after birth, remains open. An open PDA can cause significant respiratory problems and heart failure. In this case, the echocardiogram revealed a small PDA, but it was not hemodynamically significant, and we decided to manage it conservatively with close monitoring.

Days turned into weeks, and the patient remained on respiratory support. We gradually weaned the $FiO_2$ and ventilator settings as the lung function improved. The transition from mechanical ventilation to CPAP, and eventually to high-flow nasal cannula, was a slow and cautious process, ensuring that the patient could maintain adequate oxygenation and ventilation at each step.

Throughout this period, the multidisciplinary team played a crucial role. Neonatologists, respiratory therapists, nurses, and nutritionists collaborated to provide comprehensive care. Regular family meetings were held to update the parents on the patient's progress and to provide emotional support during this stressful time.

The patient showed remarkable resilience. By the end of the third week, the respiratory status had significantly improved. The need for respiratory support diminished, and the patient was able to breathe independently for short periods. The chest X-rays showed almost clear lungs, a testament to the effectiveness of the surfactant therapy and the meticulous care provided.

As the patient's respiratory function stabilized, we focused on optimizing nutrition and growth. Enteral feeding was increased, and the nasogastric tube was eventually removed as the patient demonstrated the ability to feed orally. Weight gain, though slow, was steady, and the overall clinical status was stable.

Finally, after six weeks in the NICU, the patient was ready for discharge. The journey had been long and fraught with challenges, but the outcome was positive. The patient was breathing independently, growing steadily, and showing no signs of the major complications that we had vigilantly monitored for.

# CHAPTER SIX

## BRADYCARDIA

AS I STOOD in the brightly lit Neonatal Intensive Care Unit (NICU), the rhythmic beeping of monitors provided a constant reminder of the fragile lives under my care. The sterile scent of antiseptic was ever-present, a subtle reassurance of the cleanliness and precision required in this delicate environment. The NICU was a place of extremes, where the smallest of patients fought the biggest battles, and every decision carried immense weight.

The patient, born prematurely at 32 weeks, had been admitted to our unit shortly after birth. He was tiny, weighing just under three pounds, with translucent skin and delicate limbs. Despite his early arrival, he had initially shown signs of resilience. However, on his second day of life, the situation took a drastic turn. The monitors began to show frequent episodes of brady-cardia—an abnormally slow heart rate for his age and size.

Bradycardia in neonates is not uncommon, but in a premature infant, it is a cause for significant concern. The patient's heart rate often dropped below 80 beats per minute, alarming the NICU team. Our immediate task was to stabilize him and understand the underlying cause of these episodes.

The first step was a comprehensive assessment. We initiated continuous electrocardiogram (ECG) moni-toring to keep a close watch on his heart rhythm. Blood samples were taken to check for electrolyte imbalances, infection, and other metabolic disturbances. An echocar-diogram was performed to visualize the structure and function of his heart, ensuring there were no congenital abnormalities contributing to his condition.

The initial blood work revealed mild metabolic acidosis, a common finding in preterm infants but not severe enough to explain the bradycardia. The echocar-diogram showed a structurally normal heart, which was a relief. However, the ECG revealed intermittent episodes of heart block, where the electrical signals from the atria to the ventricles were delayed or blocked entirely.

Given these findings, we developed a detailed treat-

ment plan. The primary goal was to manage the bradycardia episodes while addressing any underlying issues
that could be contributing to his condition.

Firstly, we started the patient on a continuous infusion of dopamine. Dopamine is a catecholamine that acts
on the heart to increase its rate and improve cardiac
output. We carefully titrated the dose, starting at 5
micrograms per kilogram per minute, gradually
increasing it until we saw a stable heart rate above 100
beats per minute. This required close monitoring of
blood pressure and heart rate, adjusting the infusion rate
as needed.

In addition to dopamine, we administered intravenous fluids to ensure adequate hydration and maintain
electrolyte balance. We used a combination of saline and
dextrose solutions, tailored to his needs based on regular
blood tests. Electrolytes such as potassium and calcium
were closely monitored and supplemented as necessary,
as imbalances could exacerbate bradycardia.

Antibiotics were also started empirically to cover the
possibility of neonatal sepsis, a common cause of bradycardia in premature infants. We used a broad-spectrum
antibiotic regimen, including ampicillin and gentamicin,
while awaiting the results of blood cultures. Fortunately,
the cultures returned negative after 48 hours, allowing
us to discontinue the antibiotics.

Despite these interventions, the patient continued to experience intermittent bradycardia, particularly during periods of feeding and handling. We suspected that these episodes were triggered by vagal stimulation, a common occurrence in preterm infants due to their immature autonomic nervous system. To mitigate this, we minimized handling and used gentle, slow feeding techniques via a nasogastric tube to reduce the risk of vagal-induced bradycardia.

As days turned into weeks, the patient remained stable but fragile. The dopamine infusion helped maintain his heart rate, but we knew this was not a long-term solution. Our neonatology team, in consultation with pediatric cardiologists, decided to initiate oral caffeine citrate therapy. Caffeine is a well-known stimulant of the central nervous system and has been shown to reduce episodes of apnea and bradycardia in preterm infants.

We started caffeine citrate at a loading dose of 20 milligrams per kilogram, followed by a maintenance dose of 5 milligrams per kilogram once daily. The transition from dopamine to caffeine was done gradually to ensure he remained hemodynamically stable. Over the next few days, we saw a significant reduction in the frequency and severity of bradycardia episodes.

Throughout this period, the patient's overall condition slowly improved. His weight began to increase steadily, and he showed signs of better tolerance to feeding. The caffeine therapy allowed us to wean off the dopamine completely, and his heart rate stabilized within the normal range for his gestational age.

However, our vigilance remained high. Continuous monitoring was essential, as premature infants are prone to various complications. Regular blood tests, ECGs, and echocardiograms were performed to ensure no new issues arose. We also focused on providing supportive care, including maintaining a warm environment, careful monitoring of oxygen levels, and ensuring proper nutrition.

As the patient approached what would have been his full-term gestational age, his condition had markedly improved. The episodes of bradycardia had become rare and brief, managed effectively with caffeine therapy. His weight gain was consistent, and he began to show signs of readiness for more typical neonatal care, moving towards the less intensive side of the NICU.

Finally, the day came when we could begin the transition to oral feeding. This was a critical step, as it required coordination of his suck-swallow-breathe reflex, which can be challenging for preterm infants. We started with small amounts of breast milk, carefully observing for any signs of distress or bradycardia. To our relief, he tolerated the feeds well, and his heart rate remained stable.

After several days of successful oral feeding, we prepared for his discharge from the NICU. A comprehensive care plan was developed, including instructions for follow-up appointments with neonatology and pediatric cardiology, as well as continued caffeine therapy until he reached a more mature age.

As I signed off on his discharge summary, detailing the intricacies of his NICU stay and the precise care he would need going forward, I couldn't help but feel optimistic. While the road ahead would still have challenges, the patient had overcome significant odds. The beeping of the monitors, which once signaled danger, now served as a gentle reminder of the vigilance and dedication required in the NICU—a place where the tiniest hearts fight the biggest battles and, against all odds, often emerge victorious.

# CHAPTER SEVEN

## PNEUMONIA

I'VE BEEN WORKING in the NICU for ten years and I still enter it daily with the same vigor to help these children. I see each patient as someone with a full life ahead of them and I'm there to ensure they get that chance at life. Each tiny patient in the unit represented a delicate life, fighting against the odds. Among them, one patient stood out that day—a premature infant, born at 30 weeks, who had developed a severe case of pneumonia.

The patient had been in the NICU for two weeks, having been born prematurely due to maternal complications. Initially, the infant showed signs of improvement, but over the last 48 hours, there had been a worrying decline in respiratory function. The infant was struggling, and it was clear that immediate and intensive intervention was required.

Upon examining the patient, I noted the rapid and labored breathing, with grunting and nasal flaring—a sign of respiratory distress. The oxygen saturation levels were dangerously low, despite being on supplemental oxygen. The patient's skin had a bluish tint, indicative of cyanosis. A chest X-ray revealed a telltale pattern of diffuse infiltrates, confirming the diagnosis of pneumonia. The lungs were filled with fluid and pus, making it incredibly difficult for the patient to breathe.

The first step in our treatment plan was to ensure adequate oxygenation. The patient was already on nasal CPAP (Continuous Positive Airway Pressure), but it was no longer sufficient. We made the decision to intubate the patient and initiate mechanical ventilation to support the failing respiratory system. Intubation was performed swiftly and carefully, and the ventilator settings were adjusted to ensure optimal oxygen delivery while minimizing the risk of further lung injury.

Next, we needed to address the infection. Blood cultures and a tracheal aspirate were taken to identify the causative organism. In the meantime, we started the patient on broad-spectrum antibiotics, given the urgency of the situation. The initial antibiotic regimen included ampicillin and gentamicin, both administered intravenously. These antibiotics were chosen for their effectiveness against common neonatal pathogens, including Group B Streptococcus and Escherichia coli.

Fluids and nutrition were also crucial aspects of the treatment plan. The patient was already receiving parenteral nutrition due to prematurity, but we had to be cautious with fluid management. Overhydration could worsen the pulmonary edema, while underhydration could compromise perfusion and organ function. We carefully calculated the fluid requirements and adjusted the intravenous fluid rate accordingly, monitoring the patient's urine output and electrolytes closely.

The patient's immune system was underdeveloped, and additional support was necessary. We administered intravenous immunoglobulins (IVIG) to help bolster the infant's immune response. IVIG can be beneficial in fighting infections in immunocompromised patients, and we hoped it would give the patient a fighting chance.

Monitoring the patient's progress was critical. We performed regular arterial blood gas analyses to assess the effectiveness of ventilation and oxygenation. The results guided our adjustments to the ventilator settings. Frequent chest X-rays were taken to monitor the progression or resolution of the pneumonia. We also tracked inflammatory markers, such as C-reactive protein (CRP) and white blood cell counts, to gauge the response to antibiotics.

The patient's condition remained precarious. Despite our interventions, the infant continued to struggle. We considered the possibility of a more resistant organism or a viral co-infection. Given the lack of immediate improvement, we expanded the antibiotic coverage to include vancomycin and cefotaxime, targeting potential methicillin-resistant Staphylococcus aureus (MRSA) and other resistant bacteria.

Supportive care was equally important. We ensured that the patient was kept warm and comfortable, with minimal handling to reduce stress. Pain and sedation management were essential, as the ventilator and other interventions could cause significant discomfort. We used a combination of fentanyl and midazolam for pain relief and sedation, carefully titrating the doses to balance comfort and respiratory drive.

The following days were a tense and continuous battle. The patient's vital signs fluctuated, and there were moments of profound desaturation that required immediate intervention. We adjusted the ventilator settings frequently, oscillating between high-frequency ventilation and conventional ventilation as needed. Surfactant therapy was also administered to improve lung compliance and reduce the work of breathing.

On the fourth day of intensive treatment, there was a slight but hopeful improvement. The patient's oxygenation levels stabilized, and the blood gases showed better pH and carbon dioxide levels. The repeat chest X-ray indicated a reduction in infiltrates, suggesting that the antibiotics were starting to take effect. Encouraged by these signs, we continued with the current treatment plan, maintaining close surveillance.

By the end of the first week, the patient's condition had significantly improved. The oxygen requirements decreased, and we were able to gradually wean the ventilator settings. The blood cultures came back, identifying the causative organism as Klebsiella pneumoniae, a gram-negative bacterium. Fortunately, the chosen antibiotics were effective against this pathogen, and we continued the full course of treatment.

Nutrition remained a priority as the patient's condition stabilized. We transitioned from parenteral nutrition to enteral feeding, starting with small amounts of expressed breast milk delivered through a nasogastric tube. The patient tolerated the feeds well, and we gradually increased the volume, ensuring adequate caloric intake to support growth and recovery.

Throughout this period, the patient's progress was a testament to the resilience of premature infants and the effectiveness of a comprehensive treatment plan. The infection markers normalized, and the inflammatory response subsided. The patient's lungs continued to clear, and the respiratory effort lessened.

Finally, after two weeks of intensive treatment, the patient was extubated and placed back on nasal CPAP, followed by high-flow nasal cannula oxygen. The transition was smooth, and the patient continued to breathe comfortably. The improvement in respiratory function was remarkable, and the patient began to gain weight steadily.

As the days passed, the patient's need for supplemental oxygen decreased, and the feeding volume increased. The recovery was slow but steady. The follow-up chest X-rays showed clear lungs, and the blood tests confirmed the resolution of the infection. The patient had overcome a significant hurdle, emerging from a critical illness with a promising outlook.

While the patient's journey in the NICU was far from over, the resolution of pneumonia marked a significant milestone. The collaborative effort and relentless dedication to providing the best possible care had paid off.

In the NICU, every story is unique, every life precious. The patient's case was a stark reminder of the critical importance of early detection and aggressive treatment. The road ahead would still be long, but for now, the patient had overcome one of the toughest battles, and that was a victory worth celebrating.

# CHAPTER EIGHT

## COARCTATION OF THE AORTA

THE NIGHT I first encountered the patient was one of those long, dragging nights in the NICU where every second seemed to stretch into eternity. I was just finishing up with a routine check on another newborn when the call came in from the ER. They had a neonate in distress, showing signs of severe respiratory difficulty and poor feeding. The baby had been born just hours earlier and was already in critical condition. The team quickly prepared a space for the new arrival.

The patient was wheeled into the NICU in an incubator, a tiny, fragile being connected to a multitude of tubes and wires. Their skin was a dusky blue, a clear sign of inadequate oxygenation, and they were grunting with every breath, struggling to get enough air. The nurses swiftly moved the patient to the warmer, and I began my initial assessment.

Listening to the heart, I noted a distinct murmur, a telltale sign that something was amiss with the baby's cardiovascular system. The pulses in the lower extremities were weak and almost imperceptible, further suggesting a significant cardiac anomaly. The patient's oxygen saturation levels were dangerously low despite supplemental oxygen. We needed to act quickly.

I ordered an echocardiogram, which confirmed my suspicions: the patient had Coarctation of the Aorta (CoA). This congenital heart defect involves a narrowing of the aorta, the major artery that carries blood from the heart to the rest of the body. The narrowing was severe, causing a significant obstruction to blood flow. The left ventricle was under tremendous pressure, struggling to pump blood through the constricted aorta, which was leading to the patient's critical condition.

The treatment plan for CoA in such a young patient is intricate and requires meticulous planning and execution. We needed to stabilize the patient before any surgical intervention could be considered. The first step was to administer prostaglandin E1 (PGE1) to keep the ductus arteriosus open. This ductus is a normal fetal blood vessel that usually closes soon after birth. By keeping it open, we could temporarily allow blood to bypass the narrowed section of the aorta, improving oxygenation and perfusion to the lower half of the body.

I prescribed an infusion of PGE1 at a starting dose of 0.05 mcg/kg/min, carefully titrating to maintain the ductus arteriosus patency. The patient was also placed on inotropic support with a low dose of dopamine at 5 mcg/kg/min to improve cardiac output and support blood pressure. Additionally, I initiated mechanical ventilation to ensure adequate oxygenation and to reduce the work of breathing.

As the PGE1 infusion began, I monitored the patient closely for signs of improvement. Over the next few hours, there was a slight but noticeable increase in oxygen saturation levels, and the patient's color started to improve from the dusky blue to a more acceptable pinkish hue. However, the patient remained critically ill, and I knew that this was just the first step.

The next morning, after a long night of vigilant monitoring and adjustment of medications, the cardio-thoracic surgical team arrived for a consultation. Given the severity of the CoA, they agreed that surgery was necessary and urgent. The plan was to perform a resection of the narrowed segment of the aorta with an end-to-end anastomosis. This procedure involves cutting out the narrowed section and directly connecting the two healthy ends of the aorta.

Preoperatively, I continued to manage the patient's condition with the PGE$_1$ infusion and inotropic support, along with careful fluid management to avoid fluid overload, which could exacerbate heart failure. The patient was closely monitored for any signs of deterioration. The surgical team and I discussed the risks and benefits of the surgery with the patient's parents, ensuring they understood the gravity of the situation.

The day of the surgery, the patient was transported to the operating room under the vigilant care of our transport team. I accompanied them, ensuring that the PGE$_1$ infusion was uninterrupted and that all vital parameters were stable. The surgical team took over, and I returned to the NICU to continue caring for our other patients, anxiously awaiting updates from the OR.

After several hours, I received the news that the surgery was successful. The narrowed segment of the aorta had been resected, and the ends were successfully reconnected. The patient was stable and being transferred back to the NICU for postoperative care.

Postoperatively, the focus was on maintaining hemodynamic stability and preventing complications. The patient remained on mechanical ventilation, and I adjusted the ventilator settings to gradually wean off support as their respiratory status improved. The PGE$_1$

infusion was tapered and eventually discontinued as the repaired aorta was now allowing adequate blood flow.

Pain management was crucial, so I prescribed a regimen of analgesics, including a continuous infusion of fentanyl at 1 mcg/kg/hr, adjusted as needed based on the patient's response. I also started a course of broad-spectrum antibiotics, such as cefotaxime, to prevent any postoperative infections, which are a significant risk in such delicate patients.

Over the next several days, the patient showed signs of steady improvement. The oxygen saturation levels remained stable, and the arterial blood gases were within acceptable ranges. The heart murmur was now less pronounced, indicating improved blood flow through the aorta. The patient's lower extremities were warmer, and the pulses were stronger and more palpable.

Feeding was another critical aspect of the postoperative care plan. Initially, the patient received total parenteral nutrition (TPN) to ensure adequate caloric intake without putting stress on the newly repaired aorta. Gradually, as the patient's condition stabilized, we introduced small amounts of enteral feeding through a nasogastric tube, monitoring closely for any signs of feeding intolerance.

I continued to monitor the patient for any signs of complications, such as re-coarctation, infection, or issues related to the surgery itself. The echocardiograms performed postoperatively showed good function of the heart and no significant gradient across the repair site, which was encouraging.

After about two weeks in the NICU, the patient was stable enough to begin the weaning process from mechanical ventilation. This process was done gradually, ensuring that the patient could maintain adequate respiratory function without assistance. Once the patient was successfully extubated, we continued to monitor their respiratory status, providing supplemental oxygen as needed.

Throughout this period, the patient's condition continued to improve. The cardiovascular status remained stable, and the patient began to gain weight steadily, an important indicator of overall health and recovery. By the end of the third week, the patient was on full enteral feeds and no longer required inotropic support. The patient's progress was remarkable, considering the critical condition at presentation.

As the patient's condition continued to stabilize, the time came to prepare for discharge from the NICU. This process involved detailed coordination with the pediatric cardiologist who would follow the patient's long-term care. I prepared a comprehensive discharge summary, outlining the initial presentation, the critical care interventions, surgical details, and the postoperative management plan.

The day the patient left the NICU was a moment of immense satisfaction and relief. Seeing a tiny, fragile life that had been at the brink of death recover and grow stronger was a profound reminder of why we do what we do. The journey was far from over for the patient, but the most critical phase had been successfully navigated.

I watched as the parents, who had been steadfast and hopeful throughout the ordeal, gently picked up their baby, now pink and breathing comfortably, and left the NICU. This moment, filled with a mix of exhaustion and fulfillment, was a testament to the resilience of the human spirit and the advancements in medical science that make such recoveries possible.

The patient's recovery was a team effort, involving the expertise and dedication of nurses, surgeons, respiratory therapists, and many others.

# CHAPTER NINE

## GASTROSCHISIS

THE PATIENT WAS BROUGHT IN SHORTLY after birth, a tiny, fragile newborn born with a condition known as gastroschisis. This rare congenital defect, characterized by the intestines protruding outside the abdomen through a hole next to the belly button, required immediate and meticulous care.

The initial diagnosis was made based on prenatal ultrasounds, which showed the exposed intestines floating in the amniotic fluid. The moment the patient arrived, the severity of the condition was evident. The exposed organs were at high risk for infection and damage, and the priority was to stabilize the patient and prepare for surgical intervention.

First, we assessed the extent of the protrusion. The intestines were not only outside the abdominal cavity but also appeared swollen and inflamed. The patient was at high risk of dehydration and heat loss due to the exposed tissues. We quickly placed the intestines in a sterile, transparent plastic bag to protect them and minimize fluid loss while maintaining sterility. The bag was gently secured around the defect to prevent any additional trauma to the delicate tissues.

Next, we focused on stabilizing the patient's vital signs. The patient was placed in an incubator to maintain body temperature, and an intravenous (IV) line was inserted to administer fluids, electrolytes, and antibiotics. The antibiotics were crucial to prevent any infection, given the direct exposure of the intestines to the external environment. We used a broad-spectrum antibiotic regimen, typically including ampicillin and gentamicin, to cover a wide range of potential pathogens.

While the patient was being stabilized, a multidisciplinary team, including pediatric surgeons, neonatologists, and anesthesiologists, convened to plan the surgical repair. The goal was to return the intestines to the abdominal cavity and close the defect. However, given the swelling and inflammation of the intestines, it was clear that a single-stage closure might not be possible.

The patient was taken to the operating room for the first surgery. The surgeons performed a careful inspection and gently attempted to place the intestines back into the abdomen. However, due to the swelling, only a portion of the intestines could be returned without causing excessive pressure on the abdominal cavity, which could compromise respiratory and circulatory function. A silo, a special sterile pouch, was placed over the remaining exposed intestines. This allowed for gradual reduction of the intestines back into the abdomen over the next few days.

Post-operatively, the patient was returned to the NICU for close monitoring. Pain management was a critical aspect of care, and the patient was given analgesics, including morphine, to ensure comfort. Nutritional support was provided through total parenteral nutrition (TPN), a method of feeding that bypasses the gastrointestinal tract by delivering nutrients directly into the bloodstream. This was essential as the patient's intestines needed time to recover and were not ready for enteral feeding.

Over the next few days, the silo was gradually tightened to encourage the intestines to move back into the abdominal cavity. This process required careful monitoring for signs of distress or complications such as bowel obstruction or compromised blood flow to the intestines. Each day, the patient showed resilience, tolerating the gradual reduction process without significant issues.

After several days, the patient was taken back to the

operating room for the final surgery to close the abdominal defect. This time, the intestines had reduced enough to allow for complete closure. The surgeons performed a primary closure of the defect, ensuring that the abdominal cavity could accommodate the intestines without excessive pressure.

Back in the NICU, the focus shifted to recovery and monitoring for potential complications. The patient was closely observed for signs of infection, bowel function, and overall healing. The surgical site was kept clean and sterile, with dressings changed regularly. We continued the antibiotic regimen to minimize the risk of postoperative infection.

As the patient's condition stabilized, we gradually introduced minimal enteral feeding, starting with small amounts of breast milk or formula through a nasogastric tube. This transition was done cautiously to ensure that the intestines could handle the introduction of food without causing complications such as feeding intolerance or necrotizing enterocolitis, a severe intestinal infection.

Day by day, the patient showed signs of improvement. The intestines began to function more effectively, and we were able to gradually increase the volume and frequency of feedings. The TPN was slowly reduced as enteral feeding became more established. The patient tolerated these changes well, and we monitored weight gain and overall growth closely.

Throughout this period, we provided supportive care, including respiratory support with oxygen as needed and regular assessments of vital signs. The patient's pain was managed effectively, and we monitored for any signs of discomfort or distress.

One of the most critical aspects of care was monitoring for complications associated with gastroschisis and its repair. We conducted regular abdominal ultrasounds and X-rays to ensure that there were no issues such as bowel obstruction or perforation. Blood tests were done frequently to check for signs of infection, electrolyte imbalances, and overall nutritional status.

After several weeks in the NICU, the patient's condition continued to improve. The surgical site healed well, and there were no signs of infection or other complications. The patient began to thrive, gaining weight and showing normal developmental progress for a newborn.

Finally, after a long and challenging journey, the patient was ready to be discharged from the NICU. The transition to home care was carefully planned, with detailed instructions provided to the family regarding feeding, medication administration, and follow-up appointments. The patient would need ongoing moni-

toring and care from a pediatric surgeon and gastroen-
terologist to ensure continued growth and development.

Though the NICU journey ended successfully for
this patient, I knew that their medical journey was far
from over. They would continue to need specialized care
and monitoring, but the progress made in those early
weeks was a critical foundation for a healthier future.

# CHAPTER TEN

## HYPOGLYCEMIA

MY DAY BEGAN with the rounds, reviewing the status of each tiny patient under our care. It wasn't long before I was called to a new case – a newborn who had been admitted just hours earlier.

The patient was born prematurely at 34 weeks and weighed a mere 1.8 kilograms. The baby was transferred to our NICU from the delivery room after exhibiting signs of distress. As I reviewed the initial assessments, it was clear that the baby had hypoglycemia, a condition where the blood sugar levels are dangerously low. This can be a critical condition for newborns, especially preterm ones, as their ability to regulate glucose levels is not fully developed.

The initial blood glucose level was alarmingly low at 20 mg/dL (normal levels for newborns should be between 40-60 mg/dL). The attending nurse had already initiated an intravenous (IV) glucose infusion to stabilize the baby, but I needed to ensure a comprehensive treatment plan was in place.

I ordered a bolus of 10% dextrose at a dose of 2 mL/kg, which equated to 3.6 mL for our patient. This initial intervention was crucial to quickly elevate the glucose levels and prevent any potential complications such as seizures or brain damage. After the bolus, we continued with a continuous infusion of 10% dextrose at a rate of 6 mg/kg/min, gradually tapering to 5 mg/kg/min once stabilization was observed.

While the immediate response to the dextrose bolus was promising, it was essential to identify the underlying cause of the hypoglycemia. Premature infants often have low glycogen stores and immature liver function, but other potential causes needed to be ruled out. I ordered a series of blood tests, including a comprehensive metabolic panel, serum insulin levels, cortisol, growth hormone, and a critical sample during hypoglycemia to measure ketone bodies and free fatty acids.

The metabolic panel revealed slightly elevated liver enzymes, which wasn't unusual for a preterm infant but required monitoring. Serum insulin levels were within normal limits, ruling out hyperinsulinism as a cause. Cortisol and growth hormone levels were also normal, suggesting that adrenal insufficiency and growth hormone deficiency were unlikely contributors. The critical sample showed low ketone bodies, which indicated that the baby's body was not producing enough glucose from fat stores – a sign of impaired gluconeogenesis.

With these results, I concluded that the primary cause of the hypoglycemia was the combination of prematurity and insufficient glycogen stores. The patient's liver simply wasn't mature enough to maintain normal glucose levels independently.

Next, I focused on ensuring the baby received adequate nutrition to support growth and stabilize glucose levels. Breast milk is the ideal source of nutrition for newborns, but in this case, the baby's immature digestive system made it challenging. I consulted with the nutritionist and decided on a feeding regimen that included fortified breast milk through a nasogastric tube. The fortification provided additional calories and essential nutrients while being gentle on the baby's digestive system.

We began with small volumes of 10 mL every two hours, closely monitoring the blood glucose levels before and after each feeding. The gradual increase in enteral feeds was essential to transition the baby from IV to oral nutrition without causing fluctuations in blood sugar levels.

The initial response to the feeding regimen was positive. Blood glucose levels stabilized within the first 48 hours, allowing us to gradually reduce the rate of the dextrose infusion. By the end of the first week, the patient was tolerating increased volumes of fortified breast milk, and the IV glucose was discontinued. However, constant vigilance was required as preterm infants are prone to recurrent episodes of hypoglycemia.

During the second week, I observed a concerning trend. The patient's blood glucose levels occasionally dipped below 40 mg/dL, despite adequate feeding. This prompted a re-evaluation of the feeding strategy and a possible increase in caloric intake. I increased the fortification of the breast milk and included medium-chain triglyceride (MCT) oil to boost calorie density without increasing volume, which could overwhelm the baby's immature gastrointestinal system.

Additionally, I implemented a protocol for frequent, small feedings every 1.5 to 2 hours, aiming to maintain a steady supply of glucose. This approach required meticulous coordination with the nursing staff to ensure timely feedings and glucose monitoring.

The patient's overall condition showed gradual improvement. Weight gain was steady, reaching 2.1 kilograms by the third week. This weight gain was a positive indicator of the baby's overall health and metabolic stability. However, the occasional dips in blood glucose levels necessitated ongoing monitoring and adjustments to the feeding regimen.

To support long-term glucose homeostasis, I introduced oral glucose gel as an immediate intervention for any hypoglycemic episodes. This gel, applied inside the cheek, provided a quick source of glucose while we adjusted the feeding plan.

As the fourth week approached, the patient's blood glucose levels had stabilized significantly, with fewer instances of hypoglycemia. The consistent feeding schedule, combined with fortified breast milk and MCT oil, proved effective. By now, the baby had reached 2.4 kilograms, a notable improvement from the initial admission weight.

The baby's clinical progress was encouraging. The team and I decided it was time to slowly transition the patient to on-demand breastfeeding while continuing supplemental fortified feeds. This transition required careful planning to ensure the baby could maintain adequate glucose levels without the controlled environment of scheduled feedings.

The patient adapted well to on-demand breastfeeding, a promising sign of both developmental maturity and metabolic stability. I continued to monitor glucose levels, though the frequency of testing was gradually reduced as stability was demonstrated. The last week in the NICU was marked by the baby's ability to maintain normal glucose levels independently, a milestone that indicated readiness for discharge planning.

Upon discharge, the patient weighed 2.6 kilograms and had consistently normal glucose levels. The detailed discharge plan included continued fortified feeds and frequent follow-ups with the pediatrician and nutritionist to ensure ongoing growth and metabolic health.

The patient's successful recovery and transition to outpatient care underscored the importance of personalized treatment plans, continuous monitoring, and the adaptability required in neonatal medicine.

PUBLISHER'S EXCERPT
DIAGNOSIS: RARE MEDICAL CASES: VOLUME 1

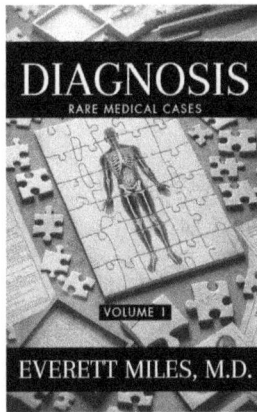

## Megaesophagus

When I first saw the patient, his chief complaints were consistent with severe dysphagia and regurgitation. These symptoms are hallmark presentations of esophageal motility disorders. Dysphagia, the sensation of difficulty swallowing, can be classified as either oropharyngeal or esophageal. The patient's history suggested esophageal dysphagia, given the sensation of food getting stuck in the lower chest area.

The patient's presentation led me to suspect achalasia, an esophageal motility disorder characterized by the failure of the LES to relax and the absence of esophageal peristalsis. The pathophysiology of achalasia involves the degeneration of the myenteric plexus, particularly affecting the inhibitory neurons responsible for the relaxation of the LES. The exact etiology remains unclear, but it is thought to involve autoimmune mechanisms, viral infections, or genetic predispositions.

To confirm the diagnosis, I ordered a barium swallow study. This radiographic examination involves the patient swallowing barium sulfate, a contrast medium, which then coats the lining of the esophagus and allows for detailed X-ray imaging. The classic finding of a "bird-beak" appearance at the gastroesophageal junction, along with a dilated esophagus, was evident in our patient. This appearance results from the narrowed LES and the dilated proximal esophagus due to retained food and secretions.

Next, an esophagogastroduodenoscopy (EGD) was performed. EGD allows direct visualization of the esophageal mucosa and can rule out other potential causes of dysphagia, such as malignancies, strictures, or eosinophilic esophagitis. In this patient, the EGD confirmed a markedly dilated esophagus with retained food particles but no obstructive lesions or mucosal abnormalities.

The definitive diagnostic test for achalasia is esophageal manometry. This test measures the pressure dynamics within the esophagus and LES. Our patient's manometry findings showed an elevated resting pressure of the LES, incomplete relaxation of the LES during swallowing, and aperistalsis in the esophageal body. These findings are diagnostic of type II achalasia, characterized by pan-esophageal pressurization and preserved residual pressure at the LES.

Once the diagnosis was confirmed, we discussed various treatment options with the patient. The primary aim of treatment in achalasia is to reduce LES pressure to facilitate esophageal emptying and relieve symptoms. Treatment options include:

1. Pneumatic Dilation: This involves endoscopic insertion of a balloon that is inflated to disrupt the LES muscle fibers. It is effective but carries a risk of esophageal perforation.

2. Surgical Myotomy: The Heller myotomy

involves cutting the LES muscle fibers to reduce pressure. It can be performed laparoscopically and is often combined with a fundoplication to prevent reflux.

3. Pharmacologic Therapy: Medications such as nitrates or calcium channel blockers can temporarily reduce LES pressure but are often not sufficient for severe cases.

4. Botulinum Toxin Injection: Endoscopic injection of botulinum toxin into the LES can temporarily reduce LES pressure but requires repeated treatments and is generally reserved for patients who are not surgical candidates.

Given the patient's relatively good health and the severity of his symptoms, we opted for a laparoscopic Heller myotomy with partial fundoplication. This approach offered a high success rate and long-term symptom relief.

The patient underwent preoperative assessments to ensure he could tolerate the procedure. These assessments included complete blood counts, metabolic panels, chest X-ray, and ECG. All results were within normal limits, and he was cleared for surgery.

The laparoscopic Heller myotomy was performed under general anesthesia. The procedure involved five small abdominal incisions through which a laparoscope and surgical instruments were inserted. The esophagus was carefully mobilized, and the muscle fibers of the LES were cut longitudinally, extending onto the gastric cardia. This myotomy effectively reduced the LES pressure, allowing easier passage of food into the stomach.

To prevent postoperative gastroesophageal reflux, a partial fundoplication (Dor fundoplication) was performed. This involves wrapping the fundus of the stomach around the posterior aspect of the esophagus to create a valve mechanism that reduces the risk of reflux.

The surgery was completed without complications. The patient was transferred to the recovery unit for postoperative monitoring. His vital signs remained stable, and he showed steady improvement. He was initially kept on a clear liquid diet and gradually advanced to a soft diet over the following days. His symptoms of dysphagia and regurgitation resolved remarkably, and he began to regain weight.

The patient was discharged on postoperative day five with instructions to follow a modified diet and avoid strenuous activities for several weeks. At his two-week follow-up appointment, he reported significant improvement in his quality of life. He had no difficulty swallowing, and his nutritional status was improving.

A repeat barium swallow study confirmed a patent

gastroesophageal junction with good passage of contrast into the stomach, indicating successful myotomy. Over the next six months, the patient continued to do well. He adhered to dietary modifications and followed up regularly to monitor for potential complications, such as GERD.

Postoperative complications of Heller myotomy can include gastroesophageal reflux, esophageal perforation, and persistent dysphagia. Our patient developed mild gastroesophageal reflux, managed with proton pump inhibitors (PPIs). He was advised on lifestyle modifications, such as elevating the head of the bed, avoiding late meals, and limiting foods that trigger reflux.

At each follow-up visit, we monitored his progress and adjusted his treatment as needed. His weight steadily increased, and his nutritional status normalized. He experienced occasional mild chest discomfort, which we attributed to esophageal spasms and managed with calcium channel blockers. These symptoms gradually resolved over time.

The long-term prognosis for patients with achalasia treated with Heller myotomy is generally favorable. Most patients experience significant symptom relief and improved quality of life. However, long-term follow-up is essential to monitor for potential complications, such as the development of esophageal carcinoma, which has a higher incidence in patients with long-standing achalasia.

Our patient's outcome was positive. At his one-year follow-up, he remained symptom-free, with no recurrence of dysphagia or regurgitation. His nutritional status was excellent, and he had regained his pre-illness weight. Surveillance endoscopy performed at one year showed no evidence of mucosal abnormalities or Barrett's esophagus, a condition that can develop due to chronic gastroesophageal reflux.

This case of megaesophagus secondary to achalasia highlights the importance of early diagnosis and timely intervention. Achalasia, although rare, should be considered in patients presenting with progressive dysphagia and regurgitation. A thorough diagnostic approach, including barium swallow, EGD, and esophageal manometry, is essential for accurate diagnosis and classification.

The treatment of achalasia aims to relieve the obstruction at the LES and improve esophageal emptying. Laparoscopic Heller myotomy with partial fundoplication is a highly effective treatment option with durable results. Postoperative follow-up is crucial to monitor for complications and ensure long-term success.

This patient's case underscores the importance of a multidisciplinary approach involving gastroenterologists, surgeons, and dietitians to achieve optimal outcomes. Through careful evaluation, appropriate intervention, and ongoing management, patients with achalasia can achieve significant symptom relief and improved quality of life.

Reflecting on this case, I am reminded of the complexities of managing esophageal motility disorders and the critical role of individualized patient care. Each patient presents unique challenges and requires a tailored approach to achieve the best possible outcomes. This case serves as a valuable learning experience and reinforces the importance of vigilance and thoroughness in medical practice.

## DIAGNOSIS: RARE MEDICAL CASES

PUBLISHER'S EXCERPT 2
CRAZY MEDICAL STORIES: VOLUME 1

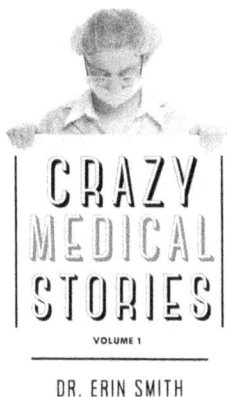

CRAZY
MEDICAL
STORIES

VOLUME 1

DR. ERIN SMITH

## Ms. Thompson's Story

Among the quiet hospital halls, amidst the hustle and
relentless march of time, certain patients' stories resonate

long after their records are filed away. One such memorable journey was with Ms. Thompson, whose case provided lessons in both the intricacies of the human body and the immense resilience of the spirit.

Ehlers-Danlos Syndrome (EDS) is a vaguely familiar term in medical circles that remains perplexing to many laypeople. Put simply, EDS comprises a group of hereditary connective tissue disorders characterized by loose joints, stretchy skin, and easy bruising. But condensing it to clinical features misses the multifaceted challenges, quiet triumphs, and touching stories interwoven through the lives affected.

Ms. Thompson's presence was an intriguing blend of delicate yet formidable. Her skin, thin and nearly translucent in its fragility, draped her slender frame with extraordinary elasticity. Her joints, hypermobile to an extreme degree, allowed a range of motion that could appear elegantly graceful. Yet these same attributes were the source of her daily tribulations.

The kaleidoscope of EDS is intricate, with the disorder spanning a spectrum rather than representing a single entity. There are numerous subtypes, each carrying distinct manifestations. Ms. Thompson's variant was the Hypermobility Type, the most common presentation. Her joints, unrestrained in their laxity, would frequently partially or completely dislocate. Even simple motions like reaching or bending carried the risk of a shoulder subluxing or a knee giving out. The very structures designed to support her body framework were profoundly unstable.

Yet the trials of EDS extend far below the surface. Lurking silently are cardiovascular, gastrointestinal, and neurological concerns. With fragile blood vessels prone to rupturing or bruising easily, even the lightest touch could elicit pain. Digestive issues like irritable bowel syndrome and gastroesophageal reflux were unwelcome companions. And then there were the headaches, a constant fierce pulsatile throbbing often arising from cervical instability due to loose neck joints.

Ms. Thompson's voluminous chart documented the myriad interventions attempted over the years to mitigate symptoms. Physical therapy was a constant, aiming to strengthen muscles surrounding hypermobile joints to provide external stability. Custom braces and splints were daily accessories, restricting motion of vulnerable joints. Finding medication regimens that balanced pain relief yet avoided side effects like gastrointestinal bleeding or medication overuse headaches was an ongoing struggle.

A particular diagnostic milestone was the arduous

quest to definitively classify her EDS subtype. With overlapping features between subtypes, EDS can be an elusive condition to conclusively categorize. For Ms. Thompson, genetic testing proved instrumental by identifying a known marker for the Hypermobility Type, eliminating guesswork. While not all EDS variants have defined genetic abnormalities, her fortunate genetic confirmation brought clarity.

As months turned to years, her story revealed both cautiously measured progress and unpredictable setbacks. With EDS' inherent volatility, even small victories were celebrated - a day without a joint dislocating, a week without digestive flares, a peaceful moment without nagging pain. But frequent regressions meant one step forward could be rapidly followed by two steps back. Patience and perspective were invaluable tools.

Yet what struck me most was not the clinical nuances of her disease, but her approach to life. EDS could have easily overshadowed everything, leaving her feeling defined by limitations. But for Ms. Thompson, it instead opened doors to new opportunities. She became an advocate, weaving her journey into a broader narrative to educate, inspire and support others on similar paths.

In her, I saw the embodiment of human resilience.

The tapestry of her life, woven with threads of hardship, endurance, hope and triumph, testified to the human capacity to not just survive, but thrive and find meaning despite adversity. Her hypermobile joints and elastic skin that were the source of pain were also symbols of her spirit's ability to bend without breaking. She became living proof that vulnerability could be transformed into strength.

As physicians, we are but witnesses to the diverse panorama of human experiences – stories that console, caution, and illuminate. Some leave ephemeral impressions, while others, like Ms. Thompson's EDS narrative, mark our hearts indelibly. Hers was a reminder that in medicine's dance between science and the soul, there are profound stories of courage, grit and unrelenting will that forever reshape our understanding of the human condition.

Ms. Thompson eventually moved closer to family, but her impact endures. When I see new EDS patients, I remember her quiet tenacity navigating relentless trials. I share her story to provide hope to families just beginning their journey with this diagnosis. Though medicine may set limited boundaries, cases like hers remind us the human spirit can still soar. Amidst life's unpredictability, we can choose how to frame our experiences - as victim or pioneer. Ms. Thompson embodied the latter, and will forever inspire me to focus on capabilities rather than limitations. Though the details may escape me, the imprint she left upon my practice never will.

## CRAZY MEDICAL STORIES

# CHAPTER ELEVEN

## INTRAVENTRICULAR HEMORRHAGE

A PREMATURE INFANT had been delivered via emergency cesarean section at 28 weeks gestation and was being rushed to our Neonatal Intensive Care Unit (NICU). As a NICU doctor, I've seen many challenging cases, but each one is unique, and this one would prove to be particularly complex.

The patient was a tiny, fragile baby, weighing just over a kilogram. The team quickly assessed the infant's condition upon arrival. The baby was in respiratory distress, requiring immediate intubation and mechanical ventilation. The first few hours were critical as we worked to stabilize the patient. Blood gas analysis revealed severe respiratory acidosis, necessitating adjustments in ventilator settings to optimize oxygenation and carbon dioxide removal.

As the hours passed, it became evident that the patient was not improving as expected. The infant's oxygen requirements remained high, and there were concerning signs of neurological instability. We decided to perform a cranial ultrasound, a standard procedure for premature infants, to check for any signs of brain injury.

The ultrasound revealed a significant finding: a Grade III intraventricular hemorrhage (IVH). Intraventricular hemorrhage is a condition where bleeding occurs inside the brain's ventricles, which can lead to increased pressure on the brain tissue and subsequent damage. IVH is a common complication in premature infants due to the fragility of their blood vessels.

The diagnosis was grim. A Grade III IVH indicated that there was blood in the ventricles and some adjacent brain tissue involvement. This type of hemorrhage can lead to long-term neurological deficits or even be life-threatening. The prognosis was uncertain, and the treatment plan needed to be comprehensive and aggressive.

Our first priority was to manage the patient's overall stability while addressing the hemorrhage. The patient was already on mechanical ventilation, so we ensured optimal ventilation and oxygenation. We closely monitored blood gases and adjusted ventilator settings as needed.

The next step was to address the potential complications of IVH. One of the most critical concerns was the possibility of post-hemorrhagic hydrocephalus, where the blood obstructs the normal flow of cerebrospinal fluid (CSF), leading to an accumulation of fluid in the brain. This can cause increased intracranial pressure and further brain damage.

To monitor for hydrocephalus, we performed daily cranial ultrasounds. Initially, there was no evidence of fluid accumulation, but we remained vigilant. We also measured the head circumference daily to detect any abnormal growth, which could indicate increasing intracranial pressure.

The patient was at high risk for seizures due to the brain injury. We started phenobarbital, an anticonvulsant medication, as a preventive measure. The dosage was carefully calculated based on the patient's weight and was administered intravenously. Continuous electroencephalogram (EEG) monitoring was initiated to detect any subclinical seizures that might not be visible through clinical observation.

Supporting the patient's cardiovascular status was also crucial. IVH can lead to instability in blood pressure and heart rate. We administered inotropic agents, specifically dopamine and dobutamine, to support the heart's function and maintain adequate blood pressure. Fluids were carefully managed to avoid fluid overload, which could exacerbate the brain swelling.

Nutrition was another vital aspect of the treatment plan. Premature infants have increased nutritional needs to support growth and development. We started parenteral nutrition through a central line, providing essential nutrients directly into the bloodstream. As the patient stabilized, we gradually introduced minimal enteral feeding with expressed breast milk, recognizing the importance of early gut priming and the immunological benefits of breast milk.

Pain management was essential, as the patient underwent numerous procedures and was in a fragile state. We used a combination of acetaminophen and, when necessary, low-dose morphine to ensure the patient was comfortable. Pain assessment in such a tiny, non-verbal patient was challenging, relying on physiological and behavioral cues.

Over the next few days, the patient's condition remained critical but stable. The daily ultrasounds showed no immediate signs of worsening hydrocephalus, but the risk was ever-present. The multidisciplinary team, including neurologists, neurosurgeons, and neonatologists, convened regularly to discuss the patient's progress and adjust the treatment plan as needed.

Despite our best efforts, the patient's neurological

status began to deteriorate. The cranial ultrasound on the seventh day revealed increasing ventricular dilation, indicative of developing hydrocephalus. The neurosurgeons were consulted, and it was decided that a temporary measure, such as a ventricular tap, would be necessary to relieve the pressure.

The ventricular tap procedure involved inserting a needle into the ventricle to drain the excess fluid and alleviate the pressure. It was a delicate procedure, given the patient's size and fragility. The neurosurgeon performed the procedure in the NICU, and we monitored the patient's response closely. The tap provided temporary relief, but it was clear that a more permanent solution might be needed if the hydrocephalus persisted.

We continued the aggressive medical management, balancing the delicate act of supporting the patient's vital functions while minimizing potential harm. The patient received meticulous care from our dedicated nursing staff, who monitored vital signs, administered medications, and provided the gentle handling that such a fragile infant required.

As days turned into weeks, the patient's condition showed signs of stabilization. The ventricular taps were performed as needed, and we carefully monitored the intracranial pressure. The patient began to tolerate enteral feeds better, and we gradually increased the volume and concentration to meet nutritional needs.

Around the third week, we noted a significant improvement. The cranial ultrasounds showed a reduction in ventricular size, indicating that the hydrocephalus was being managed effectively. The patient began to show signs of neurological improvement, with more spontaneous movements and better responses to stimuli.

However, the journey was far from over. The patient developed episodes of apnea and bradycardia, common in preterm infants but potentially exacerbated by the brain injury. We initiated caffeine citrate therapy to stimulate the respiratory centers in the brain and reduce the frequency of these episodes.

The patient also required ongoing physical therapy to support motor development and prevent complications from prolonged immobility. The physical therapists worked gently to provide passive range-of-motion exercises and positioning strategies to promote normal musculoskeletal development.

In the fourth week, we faced another challenge. The patient developed a systemic infection, likely due to the prolonged use of central lines and the invasive procedures. Blood cultures were positive for a common neonatal pathogen, and we started a broad-spectrum antibiotic regimen, later tailored based on sensitivity results. The infection caused a setback in the patient's progress, leading to increased ventilator support and closer monitoring.

Despite this setback, the patient showed remarkable resilience. The antibiotics were effective, and the infection was brought under control. The patient began to recover, and we slowly weaned off the ventilator support. The transition to non-invasive respiratory support, such as nasal CPAP, was a critical milestone in the patient's journey.

By the end of the sixth week, the patient had made significant strides. The cranial ultrasounds showed stable ventricular sizes, and the need for ventricular taps decreased. The patient was now on full enteral feeds and gaining weight steadily. The episodes of apnea and bradycardia had reduced significantly with the ongoing caffeine therapy.

Throughout this period, the patient's progress was closely monitored through a combination of clinical assessments, imaging studies, and laboratory tests. The multidisciplinary approach ensured that all aspects of the patient's care were addressed, from neurological and respiratory support to nutritional and developmental needs.

After nearly two months in the NICU, the patient

was stable enough to be transferred to a step-down unit. The journey was far from over, but the critical phase had passed. The patient would require ongoing monitoring and follow-up care to address any long-term consequences of the IVH and prematurity. The prognosis remained uncertain, with the potential for developmental delays and other complications.

The patient's journey was filled with challenges and setbacks, but also with moments of hope and progress. It reinforced the importance of a comprehensive, multidisciplinary approach to neonatal care and the incredible dedication of the healthcare team working tirelessly to give these tiny patients the best chance at life.

# CHAPTER TWELVE

## JAUNDICE

IN THE HEART of the NICU, the hum of machines and the soft cries of newborns were a constant backdrop. Among the many tiny patients, there was one who caught my attention more than the others. This particular infant was admitted with a condition we often see but never take lightly: jaundice.

The baby, born prematurely at 34 weeks, was placed in an incubator upon arrival. The yellow tint of the skin and the whites of the eyes immediately indicated hyperbilirubinemia, commonly known as jaundice. Jaundice occurs when there is a high level of bilirubin in the blood, a byproduct of the normal breakdown of red blood cells. In newborns, especially preterm ones, the liver is often not mature enough to process bilirubin efficiently.

The first step was to confirm the diagnosis through a series of blood tests. The total serum bilirubin (TSB) level was measured, and the results showed an alarming 18 mg/dL, which was dangerously high for a baby of this gestational age. It was crucial to act quickly to prevent bilirubin from crossing the blood-brain barrier and causing kernicterus, a form of brain damage.

The immediate treatment was phototherapy. The baby was placed under special blue lights, which help break down bilirubin in the skin. The lights were positioned at a safe distance to ensure maximum exposure while protecting the baby's eyes with a mask. The initial plan was to keep the baby under phototherapy continuously, with breaks only for feeding and diaper changes.

Despite our efforts, after 24 hours, the bilirubin levels remained high. The TSB level had dropped slightly to 16 mg/dL, but this was not enough. We needed a more aggressive approach. Double phototherapy was initiated, adding a second light source to increase the treatment's efficacy.

During this period, it was essential to maintain meticulous hydration and feeding schedules. Dehydration can exacerbate jaundice, so the baby was fed every two to three hours, primarily through a nasogastric tube due to the prematurity and difficulty with sucking and swallowing. The feeds consisted of expressed breast milk fortified with human milk fortifier to ensure adequate caloric and nutrient intake.

In addition to phototherapy, I monitored the baby's hydration status closely. Daily weights were taken, and fluid intake and output were meticulously recorded. An intravenous (IV) line was established to administer supplemental fluids, ensuring that the baby's electrolytes remained balanced.

As we continued with the treatment, I noticed slight improvements in the baby's condition. The skin's yellow tint was fading, and the TSB levels were gradually decreasing. However, the progress was slow, and we were not out of the woods yet.

By the third day, despite double phototherapy, the TSB level was still at 14 mg/dL. It was evident that more intensive intervention was necessary. The next step was an exchange transfusion, a procedure where the baby's blood is gradually replaced with donor blood. This procedure is risky and used only when phototherapy fails to reduce bilirubin levels sufficiently.

The procedure required careful planning and coordination. The blood bank was contacted to provide compatible donor blood, and a team of experienced nurses and a pediatric anesthesiologist were assembled. The process involved withdrawing small amounts of the baby's blood and replacing it with donor blood in a controlled manner. The goal was to reduce the bilirubin levels and remove any antibodies that might be contributing to the jaundice.

The exchange transfusion took several hours and was monitored closely for any signs of complications such as electrolyte imbalances, infection, or changes in vital signs. Thankfully, the procedure went smoothly, and the baby tolerated it well.

Post-exchange transfusion, the baby's bilirubin levels dropped significantly to 10 mg/dL. While this was still higher than we desired, it was a substantial improvement. We continued phototherapy and monitored the baby's progress with frequent blood tests.

Over the next few days, the bilirubin levels continued to decrease, and the baby's overall condition improved. The yellow tint in the skin and eyes faded, and the baby became more alert and active. The TSB levels eventually stabilized at a safe level below 8 mg/dL, allowing us to gradually wean off phototherapy.

Throughout the treatment, I was acutely aware of the importance of vigilant monitoring and timely intervention. Jaundice, while common, can quickly escalate to a life-threatening condition if not managed properly. Each decision, from initiating double phototherapy to performing the exchange transfusion, was made with careful consideration of the risks and benefits.

In addition to the medical interventions, I ensured that the parents were kept informed about their baby's condition and treatment plan. While I avoided giving them false hope, I also reassured them that we were doing everything possible to help their baby recover. The emotional toll on the parents was immense, and providing them with support and information was a critical aspect of my role.

Finally, after ten days in the NICU, the baby's condition stabilized enough for us to consider transitioning to regular care. The jaundice was under control, and the baby was feeding well and gaining weight. The yellow tint had disappeared, replaced by a healthy, pink complexion.

The baby was eventually discharged from the NICU, ready to start life outside the hospital. The journey was far from over, and continued follow-up would be necessary to monitor for any long-term effects.

# CHAPTER THIRTEEN

## NECROTIZING ENTEROCOLITIS

AS A DOCTOR SPECIALIZING in the care of the most vulnerable patients, my mornings were usually filled with the hum of incubators, the gentle beeping of monitors, and the hushed conversations of nurses and medical staff. However, that day, we received a patient who would test all our skills and knowledge: a premature infant diagnosed with Necrotizing Enterocolitis (NEC).

The patient had been born at 28 weeks' gestation, weighing just over 1,000 grams. Like many preterm infants, the patient had initially struggled with respiratory distress and required mechanical ventilation. After a few weeks, the respiratory issues stabilized, but soon after, new and troubling symptoms emerged. The baby developed abdominal distension, bloody stools, and significant lethargy. These signs pointed towards a severe gastrointestinal condition.

A series of diagnostic tests were promptly ordered. The abdominal X-ray revealed pneumatosis intestinalis, an unmistakable sign of NEC, where gas produced by bacteria accumulates in the bowel wall. This finding, coupled with the clinical symptoms, confirmed our diagnosis. The patient had developed NEC, a life-threatening condition that predominantly affects preterm infants.

Our treatment plan was aggressive. The first step was to stabilize the patient and prevent further deterioration. We immediately stopped all enteral feedings and started the patient on total parenteral nutrition (TPN) to ensure they received necessary nutrients intravenously. This would give the inflamed and infected intestines a chance to rest and heal.

Antibiotic therapy was initiated to combat the potential bacterial infection that might have triggered the NEC. The regimen included broad-spectrum antibiotics like ampicillin and gentamicin, along with metronidazole to cover anaerobic bacteria. These medications were selected based on their effectiveness in treating a broad range of bacterial infections and their known efficacy in NEC cases.

The patient was placed on a continuous positive

airway pressure (CPAP) machine to support their breathing while reducing the strain on their fragile body. Additionally, we monitored the patient's vital signs closely, ensuring that we could detect and respond to any changes immediately. Blood tests were performed regularly to check for signs of sepsis, a common and deadly complication of NEC.

Despite our efforts, the patient's condition remained critical. The abdominal distension worsened, and the baby's vital signs fluctuated wildly. It became clear that the inflammation and infection were not responding sufficiently to the conservative measures we had implemented. Surgery was becoming an unavoidable option.

A pediatric surgeon was consulted, and we discussed the best course of action. Given the severity of the patient's condition, we decided to proceed with an exploratory laparotomy. The procedure aimed to remove any necrotic sections of the bowel and to place drains if necessary to manage any abdominal abscesses.

During surgery, it was evident that a significant portion of the intestines had been affected. The surgeon carefully removed the necrotic bowel, but due to the extent of the damage, a large section had to be excised. A temporary ostomy was created to divert the stool away from the healing intestines. The hope was that, with time, the remaining healthy bowel would recover, and we could eventually reconnect the intestines in a subsequent surgery.

Postoperatively, the patient was transferred back to the NICU, where we continued intensive care. The patient remained on antibiotics to prevent any postoperative infections, and TPN was maintained to support their nutritional needs. Pain management was another critical aspect, and we used a combination of analgesics to ensure the patient remained comfortable.

The next few days were a delicate balancing act. The patient's immune system was fragile, and even a minor infection could have catastrophic consequences. Regular blood cultures and imaging studies were performed to monitor for any signs of infection or complications. The patient's condition fluctuated, with moments of hope and periods of intense concern.

As days turned into weeks, we gradually began to see signs of improvement. The patient's abdominal distension decreased, and their vital signs stabilized. The ostomy output was closely monitored, and we started to see a gradual return of bowel function. Slowly, we reintroduced minimal enteral feeding, starting with small amounts of breast milk, which is easier to digest and has protective factors that could aid in the healing process.

Nutritional support continued to be a key focus. As the patient tolerated feeds, we gradually increased the volume and caloric content, always being vigilant for any signs of feeding intolerance or recurrence of NEC. We also ensured that the patient received necessary supplements, including vitamins and minerals, to support their overall growth and development.

Throughout this period, the interdisciplinary team, including neonatologists, surgeons, nutritionists, and nurses, worked tirelessly to provide comprehensive care. Every decision was carefully weighed, considering the patient's delicate condition and the potential risks and benefits.

After several weeks of meticulous care and monitoring, the patient's condition improved significantly. The abdominal distension had resolved, and the patient was tolerating full enteral feeds. With the patient's overall stability, we scheduled the second surgery to reverse the ostomy and reconnect the intestines.

The second surgery was another critical milestone. The surgical team successfully reconnected the intestines, and the patient was closely monitored for any postoperative complications. The recovery from this second surgery was smoother than anticipated, and we saw steady progress in the patient's condition.

As the weeks passed, the patient continued to gain weight and showed no signs of recurring NEC. The transition from TPN to full enteral feeds was successful, and the patient's growth parameters improved. The patient was weaned off respiratory support and no longer required intensive monitoring for infections.

Ultimately, after several months of intensive care and multiple surgeries, the patient made a remarkable recovery. The journey had been fraught with challenges and moments of uncertainty, but the combined efforts of the entire medical team, along with the resilience of the patient, led to a positive outcome.

Although the patient's journey in the NICU came to an end, it marked the beginning of a new chapter of growth and development outside the hospital. The battle with NEC had been won, and the patient left the NICU as a symbol of hope and resilience for all of us who had cared for them.

# CHAPTER FOURTEEN

## RETINOPATHY OF PREMATURITY

I REMEMBER THE PATIENT CLEARLY, a tiny, fragile being brought into the world much too soon. Born at 26 weeks gestation, they weighed just over 800 grams, a mere whisper of life cradled in the warm, sterile environment of our NICU. As a neonatologist, the fight for every breath, every heartbeat, and every milestone was a familiar one, but each patient brought their unique battle, and this one was no exception.

The initial days were harrowing. The patient's lungs, not fully developed, required immediate and sustained support. Mechanical ventilation was essential from the first moments. Surfactant therapy was administered to reduce the surface tension in their immature lungs, allowing for more effective breathing. Every breath was a struggle, but with time, we began to see progress. The ventilator settings were gradually lowered, and eventually, we transitioned to continuous positive airway pressure (CPAP) to maintain adequate oxygenation.

At around two weeks of age, the patient started showing signs of another complication common in premature infants: Retinopathy of Prematurity (ROP). ROP is a disease that affects the blood vessels of the retina, which is the light-sensitive tissue at the back of the eye. It occurs because the blood vessels in the eyes are not fully developed at the time of birth and can grow abnormally when exposed to high levels of oxygen, as often required by premature infants.

The first indication came during a routine retinal examination. The ophthalmologist noted abnormal blood vessel growth, characteristic of stage 1 ROP, the mildest form of the disease. At this stage, the abnormal vessels are just starting to form. While it's a sign of concern, many infants' eyes can heal on their own without intervention. Despite this, we knew vigilant monitoring was crucial.

Over the next few weeks, we closely followed the patient's retinal development. The oxygen levels were meticulously controlled to balance the need for adequate systemic oxygenation while minimizing the risk of exacerbating the ROP. The patient's blood gases were checked regularly, and adjustments to the ventilator settings were made as needed.

Unfortunately, the ROP progressed to stage 2, where the abnormal blood vessels continued to grow, and there was a risk they could lead to retinal detachment. At this stage, treatment options needed to be considered more seriously. The ophthalmologist and I discussed the possibility of laser therapy, a common treatment for ROP that works by burning the peripheral areas of the retina to stop abnormal blood vessels from growing. However, we agreed to continue monitoring closely, hoping to avoid invasive procedures if possible.

At around six weeks of age, the patient's condition took a turn. The ROP advanced to stage 3, which is more severe and marked by a proliferation of abnormal blood vessels, potentially causing the retina to be pulled out of position. The decision to intervene was clear; waiting any longer could result in permanent vision loss or blindness.

We prepared the patient for laser photocoagulation therapy. The procedure involved using a laser to create small burns around the peripheral retina, which helped to slow or stop the abnormal blood vessel growth. The patient was sedated, and the procedure was performed with utmost precision and care. The burns created scars that helped to anchor the retina in place and prevent detachment.

Post-procedure, the patient was monitored closely for any signs of complications. The immediate concern was ensuring the eye did not suffer from increased inflammation or infection. Topical antibiotic and steroid eye drops were prescribed to prevent infection and reduce inflammation. These drops were administered several times a day, and the patient's eyes were examined daily to assess the healing process.

While the eyes healed, the patient's overall condition continued to improve. Their lungs became stronger, and they were eventually weaned off the ventilator and transitioned to nasal cannula oxygen support. Nutrition was another critical aspect of their care. We carefully managed their feeding regimen, starting with total parenteral nutrition (TPN) and gradually introducing enteral feeds as their gastrointestinal system matured. Breast milk, fortified with additional nutrients, was administered through a nasogastric tube, providing the essential nutrients needed for growth and development.

The weeks became months, and the patient showed remarkable resilience. The retinal examinations post-laser therapy indicated that the abnormal blood vessel growth had been effectively halted. There were no signs of further progression, and the retina remained attached, a promising outcome.

In addition to the eye care and respiratory support, we focused on the patient's overall development. Physical therapy was introduced to encourage muscle strength and coordination. Gentle, guided movements and positioning helped to promote proper musculoskeletal development. Occupational therapy was also initiated to assist with feeding and sensory integration, crucial for a premature infant's growth.

By the time the patient reached their original due date, they had made significant strides. Their respiratory needs had diminished substantially, requiring only minimal oxygen support. They had grown from a fragile 800 grams to over 2.5 kilograms, a testament to their tenacity and the comprehensive care they received.

The patient's journey in the NICU was one of numerous hurdles and small victories. Each day presented new challenges, but with the dedicated efforts of the entire medical team, the patient continued to improve. The parents were prepared for the transition to home care, and we provided detailed instructions on how to manage the patient's ongoing needs, particularly the eye care regimen.

As the NICU stay came to an end, there was a sense of achievement mixed with the understanding that the journey was far from over. The patient would require regular follow-ups with a pediatric ophthalmologist to monitor their retinal development and ensure no late-onset complications. Early intervention services were arranged to support their developmental milestones and address any delays that might arise.

The patient's story in the NICU concluded with them being discharged in a stable condition, ready to face the world outside the confines of the hospital. The scars from the laser therapy would remain, but they served as markers of a battle fought and won. The journey ahead would undoubtedly hold more chal-lenges, but the foundation laid in the NICU provided the strength to face them. In the end, the patient left the NICU not just as a survivor but as a testament to the extraordinary possibilities of modern neonatal medicine.

# CHAPTER FIFTEEN

### SEPSIS

THE NICU WAS ALWAYS a place of tension and hope, a delicate balance between life and the fragility of our smallest patients. It was within these walls that I first encountered the patient, a newborn who arrived under the most harrowing of circumstances. As I walked into the NICU that morning, I was briefed on the latest admissions and the challenges we faced.

The patient was brought in, a premature baby born at 30 weeks gestation, with a concerning history. The mother had developed chorioamnionitis during labor, a bacterial infection of the fetal membranes, which often leads to sepsis in newborns. The baby's Apgar scores were low, indicating distress at birth. Immediately, the team had to resuscitate and stabilize the infant before transferring to the NICU for intensive care.

Upon arrival, the patient was lethargic and exhibiting signs of respiratory distress. The initial examination revealed mottled skin, a concerning sign that indicated poor perfusion. The infant's heart rate was elevated, and the respiratory rate was labored. These were classic signs of sepsis, a severe infection that spreads throughout the body, overwhelming the immune system.

Sepsis in neonates, especially those born prematurely, is particularly deadly due to their underdeveloped immune systems. Our immediate priority was to confirm the diagnosis and begin aggressive treatment. Blood cultures, urine cultures, and a lumbar puncture were ordered to identify the causative organism. We also performed a chest X-ray to check for any signs of pneumonia, a common complication in septic neonates.

While awaiting the results, we initiated broad-spectrum antibiotics. The patient was started on ampicillin and gentamicin, the standard initial therapy for suspected neonatal sepsis. Ampicillin would cover Group B Streptococcus, Listeria, and enterococci, while gentamicin was aimed at Gram-negative bacteria like Escherichia coli.

We placed an umbilical venous catheter (UVC) and an umbilical arterial catheter (UAC) for administering medications and monitoring blood gases, respectively.

Intravenous fluids were started to maintain blood pressure and ensure adequate perfusion to vital organs. The patient was also placed on a ventilator to support breathing, given the respiratory distress.

The next 48 hours were critical. The patient remained under continuous monitoring, with frequent blood pressure checks, heart rate, and oxygen saturation levels. We kept a close eye on urine output to gauge kidney function, as sepsis can lead to multi-organ failure. The baby's temperature was monitored to manage any fluctuations that could indicate worsening infection or other complications.

By the second day, the blood culture results confirmed the presence of Escherichia coli, a common culprit in neonatal sepsis. This guided our antibiotic therapy more precisely. We discontinued ampicillin and continued with gentamicin, adding cefotaxime for broader coverage against Gram-negative bacteria.

The patient's condition remained tenuous. Fluid management became a balancing act to prevent both dehydration and fluid overload, which could exacerbate respiratory distress. Daily blood work was essential to monitor electrolytes, renal function, and the blood cell counts. Thrombocytopenia, or low platelet count, became a concern, and we prepared for potential platelet transfusions.

On the third day, we noted some signs of improvement. The patient's blood pressure stabilized with less need for vasopressors, medications that constrict blood vessels and increase blood pressure. Oxygen requirements decreased slightly, and there was a slight increase in spontaneous movements. However, we remained cautious, knowing that sepsis could have unpredictable courses, especially in such fragile patients.

Throughout this period, we maintained strict aseptic techniques to prevent any secondary infections. Hand hygiene, sterilized equipment, and careful handling were crucial. The patient's environment was kept as sterile as possible, with minimal handling to reduce stress and the risk of infection.

By the end of the first week, we started seeing more definitive signs of recovery. The patient's respiratory status improved enough to begin weaning off the ventilator. We switched to nasal continuous positive airway pressure (CPAP), which provided respiratory support without the invasiveness of the ventilator.

The patient's kidney function also showed signs of improvement, with urine output increasing and serum creatinine levels normalizing. We were able to reduce the intravenous fluids gradually and started enteral feeding with breast milk through a nasogastric tube.

Breast milk was chosen due to its immunological benefits and easier digestion compared to formula.

As we entered the second week, the patient continued to show signs of stabilization. Blood cultures were repeated and came back negative, indicating that the antibiotics were effective in clearing the infection. We continued the antibiotic course for the full 21 days to ensure complete eradication of the bacteria and prevent relapse.

The patient's blood counts began to normalize, and the thrombocytopenia resolved without the need for platelet transfusions. We monitored for any signs of complications such as necrotizing enterocolitis, a severe intestinal condition that can occur in premature infants, especially those recovering from sepsis. Fortunately, there were no indications of such complications.

During this time, we also assessed the patient for any potential long-term effects of the infection and the intensive treatments. Neurodevelopmental assessments were conducted to evaluate any impact on the brain, as neonatal sepsis can lead to conditions like cerebral palsy or developmental delays. Early signs were promising, but ongoing follow-up would be necessary to ensure normal development.

By the third week, the patient was off CPAP and breathing room air. Enteral feeding was well tolerated, and we gradually increased the volume and frequency. Weight gain was monitored closely, and the baby started to show healthy growth patterns.

Discharge planning began, focusing on preparing the parents for the baby's care at home. Education on signs of infection, feeding schedules, and follow-up appointments with pediatricians and specialists were part of the process. We also coordinated with social services to ensure the family had access to necessary resources and support systems.

Finally, after nearly a month in the NICU, the patient was ready to go home. The journey from the brink of death to recovery was a testament to the resilience of newborns and the tireless efforts of the NICU team. Each case like this one reinforced the importance of early recognition, aggressive treatment, and meticulous care in managing neonatal sepsis.

While the patient left the NICU, the journey was far from over. Follow-up care would be crucial in monitoring for any late-onset complications or developmental delays. The collaboration between neonatologists, pediatricians, and the family would continue to ensure the best possible outcome for the patient.

# CHAPTER SIXTEEN

## MACROSOMIA

AS A NICU DOCTOR, I've encountered numerous cases that challenged my medical knowledge and tested my emotional resilience. One such case that remains vivid in my memory involved a newborn diagnosed with macrosomia. The patient was delivered via cesarean section after a protracted labor and weighed a striking 11 pounds and 2 ounces at birth. From the moment the patient was born, it was evident that we were dealing with a complex and potentially life-threatening situation.

Macrosomia, characterized by a newborn significantly larger than average, often complicates delivery and poses numerous risks to the infant's health. The mother had gestational diabetes, which we later identified as a key contributing factor to the patient's condition. This diagnosis guided our subsequent treatment plan, which aimed to address both immediate and longer-term complications.

Upon the patient's arrival in the NICU, we initiated a thorough diagnostic assessment. The first step was to stabilize the patient's vitals. Despite the significant birth weight, the patient exhibited signs of respiratory distress, a common complication in macrosomic infants. We promptly administered oxygen and monitored the oxygen saturation levels, ensuring they remained within a safe range. The patient required continuous positive airway pressure (CPAP) to maintain adequate oxygenation due to underdeveloped lungs.

A blood glucose test revealed hypoglycemia, another frequent issue in infants of diabetic mothers. The patient's blood sugar level was alarmingly low at 35 mg/dL, necessitating immediate intervention. We administered an intravenous glucose infusion to stabilize the blood sugar levels, carefully titrating the dose to avoid fluctuations. Frequent monitoring of blood glucose levels was crucial during the first 24 hours, with adjustments made to the glucose infusion rate as needed.

The patient also underwent a comprehensive physical examination and imaging studies to identify any underlying structural anomalies or birth injuries. An abdominal ultrasound revealed hepatomegaly, an enlargement of the liver, which we attributed to excessive glycogen storage—a condition associated with maternal diabetes. This required us to closely monitor liver function tests and ensure that the liver size normalized as the patient's metabolic status stabilized.

Another pressing concern was the potential for polycythemia, a condition where the blood has an abnormally high number of red blood cells, increasing the risk of blood clots and hyperviscosity syndrome. A complete blood count confirmed an elevated hematocrit level of 68%, necessitating partial exchange transfusion to reduce the red blood cell concentration and improve circulation.

Feeding presented another challenge. Macrosomic infants often struggle with poor feeding and subsequent weight management issues. We initiated enteral feeding with expressed breast milk through a nasogastric tube, carefully monitoring the patient's tolerance and gradually increasing the volume as the patient demonstrated the ability to digest and absorb the nutrients. The patient's weight was closely monitored to ensure a steady and healthy weight gain trajectory.

Given the complexity of the patient's condition, a multidisciplinary approach was essential. We consulted with a pediatric endocrinologist to manage the metabolic aspects and a pediatric cardiologist to rule out any congenital heart defects, which are more common in macrosomic infants. An echocardiogram revealed a small ventricular septal defect, a hole in the heart's ventricular wall. While it was not immediately life-threatening, we scheduled regular follow-ups to monitor the defect's size and the patient's cardiac function.

Throughout the patient's stay in the NICU, careful attention was given to preventing infections, a significant risk factor in newborns, particularly those requiring invasive interventions. We adhered to strict aseptic techniques during all procedures and monitored for any signs of sepsis, administering prophylactic antibiotics as a precautionary measure.

The patient's progress was slow but steady. Over the course of the first week, we observed improvements in respiratory function, allowing us to gradually wean the patient off CPAP. The blood glucose levels stabilized, and the liver size reduced to within normal limits. The hematocrit levels normalized following the partial exchange transfusion, and the patient began to show signs of improved feeding tolerance.

By the end of the second week, the patient's condition had stabilized significantly. The respiratory support was discontinued, and the patient was transitioned to full oral feeds. The patient's weight gain was within expected parameters, and follow-up imaging studies showed no significant abnormalities.

Despite the initial severity of the patient's condition, the coordinated efforts of the NICU team and the multi-disciplinary specialists contributed to a successful outcome. The patient's stay in the NICU lasted a total of three weeks, during which time we addressed the acute complications of macrosomia and set the stage for a transition to outpatient care.

On discharge, the patient was in stable condition, with instructions for follow-up appointments with the pediatric endocrinologist and cardiologist to monitor the ventricular septal defect and ensure continued meta-bolic stability. The family was provided with detailed care instructions and resources to support the patient's ongoing development and health.

Ultimately, the patient's prognosis was positive, with the potential for a healthy and normal development trajectory. While the initial challenges were significant, the successful management of the patient's condition reinforced the importance of vigilance, adaptability, and the relentless pursuit of optimal outcomes in neonatal care. The experience underscored the profound impact of our work in the NICU, where every decision and intervention contributes to the delicate balance of life for our youngest and most vulnerable patients.

# CHAPTER SEVENTEEN

## PATENT DUCTUS ARTERIOSUS

AS A NEONATOLOGIST, the NICU was my second home. Each day brought new challenges and triumphs, but there was one case that lingered in my memory, a testament to the fragile strength of our tiniest patients. It was a typical Tuesday morning when I was called to assess a newborn who had been delivered prematurely at 28 weeks. The patient was a tiny, fragile being, weighing just under 1000 grams. Immediately, I could see the struggle for life in their small body, each breath a monumental effort.

The patient was initially stable but required support to breathe. We started with continuous positive airway pressure (CPAP) to help keep the lungs open. As with many preterm infants, respiratory distress syndrome was a concern, so surfactant therapy was administered shortly after birth. Despite these measures, the patient's condition remained precarious.

On the third day of life, a routine echocardiogram revealed a Patent Ductus Arteriosus (PDA). In simple terms, the ductus arteriosus is a blood vessel that allows blood to bypass the lungs in utero. Normally, it closes shortly after birth as the newborn's circulatory system transitions to breathing air. However, in preterm infants, this vessel often remains open, leading to a PDA. This can cause significant problems, including poor oxygenation and increased workload on the heart.

The echocardiogram showed a moderate-sized PDA with significant left-to-right shunting. This meant that oxygenated blood was being pushed back into the lungs rather than being circulated through the body, leading to over-circulation of the lungs and under-perfusion of the systemic organs. The patient was already showing signs of increased respiratory distress, including tachypnea and retractions, which indicated they were working harder to breathe.

Given the size of the PDA and the clinical symptoms, we decided to intervene. The first line of treatment for PDA is medical management. We started with a course of intravenous indomethacin, a nonsteroidal anti-inflammatory drug (NSAID) that helps to encourage the closure of the ductus arteriosus. Indomethacin works by inhibiting the production of prostaglandins, substances that keep the ductus open.

The patient received three doses of indomethacin over a 48-hour period. During this time, we closely monitored urine output and renal function, as indomethacin can cause reduced kidney perfusion. We also kept a close eye on the platelet count and gastrointestinal function, as NSAIDs can affect both.

After the initial course of treatment, another echocardiogram was performed. Unfortunately, it showed that the PDA had not closed completely. There was still a significant left-to-right shunt, and the patient's clinical condition had not improved as hoped. The decision was made to proceed with a second course of indomethacin.

Throughout the treatment, we provided supportive care in the NICU. The patient remained on CPAP, and we closely monitored oxygenation and ventilation. The fluid balance was meticulously managed to prevent fluid overload, which could exacerbate the PDA. Parenteral nutrition was continued to support growth and development, as the patient was not yet able to tolerate enteral feeds.

The second course of indomethacin also failed to close the PDA. At this point, the patient's respiratory distress was worsening, and they required intubation and mechanical ventilation. We initiated diuretic therapy with furosemide to help manage fluid balance and reduce pulmonary congestion. Despite these efforts, the patient's condition remained critical.

Given the failure of medical management and the patient's worsening condition, we consulted with the pediatric cardiology team to discuss surgical options. The decision was made to proceed with a PDA ligation, a surgical procedure to close the ductus arteriosus. This was not a decision taken lightly, as surgery in such a small and fragile patient carries significant risks. However, the benefits outweighed the risks, as the PDA was significantly impacting the patient's ability to oxygenate and grow.

The surgery was scheduled for the following morning. The patient was carefully prepared, and we discussed the risks and benefits with the parents, ensuring they understood the gravity of the situation. The surgical team was experienced, and we had high hopes for a positive outcome.

The PDA ligation was performed without complications. The ductus arteriosus was successfully closed, and the patient was transferred back to the NICU for postoperative care. The immediate postoperative period was critical, and we monitored for signs of bleeding, infection, and changes in hemodynamic status.

In the first 24 hours after surgery, the patient showed signs of improvement. The oxygen requirements decreased, and the mechanical ventilation settings were gradually reduced. By the third postoperative day, the patient was stable enough to be extubated and placed back on CPAP. This was a significant milestone, as it indicated that the lungs were no longer being overwhelmed by the extra blood flow from the PDA.

With the PDA closed, we could focus on the patient's growth and development. Enteral feeds were slowly introduced, starting with small amounts of breast milk through a nasogastric tube. The patient tolerated these feeds well, and we gradually increased the volume as their gut adapted. Nutrition is crucial for preterm infants, and breast milk provides not only the necessary nutrients but also protective factors that support the immature immune system.

Over the next few weeks, the patient continued to make progress. There were setbacks, as is common in the NICU, including episodes of apnea and bradycardia, which required interventions such as caffeine therapy and adjustments in respiratory support. However, the overall trend was positive.

The PDA closure allowed the heart to work more efficiently, and the patient's weight gain improved. The respiratory support was gradually weaned, and by the time the patient reached 36 weeks corrected gestational age, they were breathing on their own with minimal supplemental oxygen.

Throughout this journey, the multidisciplinary team played a crucial role. Neonatal nurses provided round-the-clock care, ensuring that the patient's needs were met and that any changes in condition were promptly addressed. Respiratory therapists managed the ventilator settings and monitored the patient's respiratory status. The pediatric cardiology team continued to follow the patient, performing regular echocardiograms to ensure there were no complications from the PDA ligation.

The day the patient was finally ready to leave the NICU was a moment of triumph. We had all invested so much in their care, and seeing them healthy and ready to go home was a reminder of why we do this work. The patient had overcome significant hurdles, and while the journey ahead would still require close follow-up and support, the worst was behind them.

———————————————

# CHAPTER EIGHTEEN

THE DAY BEGAN like any other in the NICU. I reviewed my patient list, noting the new admissions and checking on the status of ongoing cases. One patient, in particular, caught my attention—a newborn diagnosed with Pulmonary Hypertension (PH).

The patient was a preterm infant, born at 28 weeks gestation, weighing just over 1000 grams. The initial concerns at birth included respiratory distress syndrome (RDS) due to prematurity. The patient had been immediately intubated and placed on mechanical ventilation. Despite aggressive surfactant therapy and ventilation adjustments, the patient's oxygenation remained poor. An echocardiogram was performed, revealing significant pulmonary hypertension.

Pulmonary Hypertension in neonates, particularly

in preterm infants, presents a considerable challenge. It involves high blood pressure in the arteries of the lungs, leading to right ventricular dysfunction and impaired oxygenation. For this patient, the diagnosis meant a complex and multifaceted treatment plan aimed at reducing pulmonary artery pressure, improving oxygenation, and supporting the heart.

Our first line of treatment involved optimizing respiratory support. The patient was already on high-frequency oscillatory ventilation (HFOV), which is often more effective in severe PH cases compared to conventional mechanical ventilation. We aimed to keep the mean airway pressure (MAP) elevated to help maintain alveolar recruitment and improve oxygenation. The fraction of inspired oxygen ($FiO_2$) was carefully titrated to keep the patient's oxygen saturation between 92-95%, avoiding both hypoxemia and hyperoxia.

In conjunction with respiratory management, we initiated pharmacological therapy. Nitric oxide inhalation therapy was started at 20 parts per million (ppm). Nitric oxide acts as a selective pulmonary vasodilator, reducing pulmonary artery pressure without causing systemic hypotension. The patient's response to nitric oxide was closely monitored through repeated echocardiograms and blood gas analyses. Within a few hours, we noted a modest improvement in oxygenation and a slight reduction in pulmonary artery pressure.

Despite the positive initial response to nitric oxide, it became evident that the patient needed additional support. We started intravenous sildenafil, a phosphodiesterase-5 inhibitor, known to further reduce pulmonary artery pressure by enhancing the effect of nitric oxide. The initial dose was 0.35 mg/kg every 8 hours. Close monitoring was essential, as sildenafil can cause systemic hypotension. Fortunately, the patient's blood pressure remained stable, and we observed further improvement in oxygenation parameters.

The next step in our treatment plan was the careful management of fluids and nutrition. Fluid overload can exacerbate pulmonary hypertension by increasing pulmonary vascular resistance. We maintained strict fluid balance, ensuring that the patient received enough fluids to support organ function but avoiding excessive amounts. Parenteral nutrition was administered, providing essential nutrients while minimizing fluid volume. Gradually, as the patient stabilized, we introduced minimal enteral feeds to stimulate gut function.

To support the right ventricle and improve cardiac output, we started milrinone infusion. Milrinone is a phosphodiesterase-3 inhibitor that has both inotropic and vasodilatory effects, making it beneficial in managing PH. The initial loading dose was 50 micrograms/kg over 10 minutes, followed by a continuous infusion of 0.5 micrograms/kg/min. This therapy required careful monitoring of blood pressure and cardiac function.

Throughout the treatment, we faced numerous challenges. The patient's condition fluctuated, with episodes of desaturation and bradycardia. Each episode required prompt assessment and intervention. We adjusted ventilator settings, titrated medications, and ensured optimal positioning to maximize lung expansion and perfusion.

The patient showed slow but steady improvement. The frequency and severity of desaturation episodes decreased. Echocardiograms indicated a gradual reduction in pulmonary artery pressure and improved right ventricular function. We started weaning off nitric oxide, reducing the dose by 5 ppm every 12 hours while monitoring for any signs of deterioration.

By the third week, the patient had stabilized enough for us to consider transitioning from high-frequency oscillatory ventilation to conventional mechanical ventilation. This transition was done cautiously, ensuring that the patient maintained adequate oxygenation and ventilation. We continued sildenafil and milrinone, gradually tapering the doses as the patient's pulmonary pressures normalized.

Nutrition played a crucial role in the patient's recovery. Enteral feeds were slowly advanced, and we monitored for signs of feeding intolerance. The patient's weight gain was a positive indicator, suggesting good overall growth and development despite the initial critical condition.

After four weeks of intensive care, the patient reached a significant milestone. The pulmonary pressures had decreased to near-normal levels, and the right ventricular function was much improved. We successfully weaned off milrinone and later sildenafil. The patient was transitioned to nasal continuous positive airway pressure (CPAP) as the final step in respiratory support before eventual weaning to room air.

Finally, the day came when the patient no longer required respiratory support. Oxygen saturations remained stable on room air, and the echocardiogram showed no evidence of significant pulmonary hypertension. The patient was discharged from the NICU, a testament to the resilience of these tiny fighters and the dedication of the medical team.

# CHAPTER NINETEEN

### LARGE INTESTINE OBSTRUCTION

IT WAS a quiet night in the Neonatal Intensive Care Unit (NICU) when the patient was admitted. I had just completed my rounds and was looking forward to a brief respite when the call came in. The patient was a newborn, only a few hours old, transferred from a smaller hospital due to severe abdominal distension and failure to pass meconium. The referral mentioned a suspected case of large intestine obstruction, a diagnosis that required immediate attention.

Upon arrival, the patient was in a critical condition. The abdomen was notably swollen, firm to the touch, and the baby exhibited signs of distress—rapid breathing and a heart rate significantly elevated for their age. The neonate's skin had a bluish tinge, indicative of poor oxygenation, and there was notable lethargy, a concerning sign in a newborn. Immediate steps were necessary to stabilize the patient before further diagnostics could be performed.

Initial stabilization involved ensuring the patient's airway, breathing, and circulation were maintained. We placed the patient on supplemental oxygen to correct the hypoxia and inserted an intravenous line to administer fluids and medications. The first priority was to correct any electrolyte imbalances and to ensure proper hydration. Blood tests confirmed significant metabolic acidosis, a condition where the body produces too much acid or the kidneys are not removing enough acid from the body. This required careful correction with sodium bicarbonate.

With the patient stabilized, the next step was diagnostic imaging. An abdominal X-ray was performed, revealing a markedly dilated large intestine with what appeared to be a transition zone—a clear indicator of a bowel obstruction. Further imaging, specifically an ultrasound, confirmed the presence of a large intestine obstruction. The likely causes were either Hirschsprung's disease or a meconium plug syndrome, both of which are serious but treatable conditions.

Hirschsprung's disease, a congenital condition where nerve cells are missing from parts of the muscles in the bowel, seemed the most likely diagnosis. In this disease, the absence of these nerve cells means the muscles in the bowel cannot contract to move stool through the colon, leading to obstruction. The definitive diagnosis required a rectal biopsy, which we prepared to perform. This would confirm the absence of ganglion cells in the intestinal wall, solidifying our diagnosis.

The biopsy procedure was carried out under sterile conditions in the NICU. The sample obtained would take a few hours to process, but given the critical condition of the patient, we couldn't afford to wait. Immediate surgical intervention was deemed necessary to relieve the obstruction and prevent further complications such as bowel perforation or sepsis.

The patient was prepped for surgery, and with the utmost care, we transferred them to the operating room. The surgical team, experienced in neonatal procedures, took over, and I joined them to provide support and ensure continuity of care. The surgery involved a colostomy, where a section of the large intestine was brought out through the abdomen to create a stoma. This would allow waste to bypass the obstructed part of the bowel.

During the surgery, we confirmed our diagnosis. The affected segment of the intestine showed no signs of ganglion cells, consistent with Hirschsprung's disease. The obstructed segment was resected, and a colostomy was created. The surgery went smoothly, and the patient was brought back to the NICU for postoperative care.

Postoperatively, the focus was on monitoring for complications and ensuring proper recovery. The patient remained on a ventilator for the first 24 hours to support breathing and was closely monitored for signs of infection, a common risk after such procedures. Antibiotics were administered prophylactically to prevent infections. The baby's fluid and electrolyte balance was meticulously managed through intravenous infusions.

Pain management was crucial. Newborns can experience significant pain, but they often cannot express it. We administered appropriate doses of analgesics, carefully monitoring the patient for any adverse reactions. Nutritional support was also critical. Initially, the patient was fed intravenously (parenteral nutrition), providing essential nutrients directly into the bloodstream while the digestive system healed.

The rectal biopsy results returned, confirming Hirschsprung's disease. This confirmed that the initial surgical approach was correct. The patient showed signs of improvement within the first 48 hours post-surgery. The abdominal distension began to decrease, and vital signs stabilized. The skin color improved, indicating better oxygenation and circulation. By the third day, we started to see urine output increase, a positive sign that the kidneys were functioning well.

Gradually, as the patient's condition stabilized, we weaned them off the ventilator and transitioned to nasal cannula oxygen. This allowed the patient to breathe more independently while still receiving supplemental oxygen. By the end of the first week, the patient was breathing room air and showing signs of active recovery.

The colostomy required diligent care. The stoma site needed to be kept clean to prevent infection and complications. We trained the nursing staff and the patient's family in stoma care, ensuring they were comfortable and capable of managing it once the patient was ready for discharge.

The next critical phase was to monitor the patient's ability to tolerate enteral feeding. We started with minimal enteral nutrition—tiny amounts of breast milk or formula fed through a nasogastric tube. This was crucial to stimulate the bowel and ensure it was functioning correctly. Gradually, the volume of enteral feeds was increased, and we observed the patient for any signs of feeding intolerance, such as vomiting or increased abdominal distension.

Over the next few weeks, the patient's condition continued to improve. The stoma output was regular, and the patient was gaining weight, a clear indicator of good nutritional status. Regular blood tests showed normalizing electrolyte levels and a stable metabolic profile. We closely monitored the patient for any signs of Hirschsprung-associated enterocolitis, a severe and potentially life-threatening complication, but fortunately, there were no such signs.

After several weeks in the NICU, the patient was stable enough for the next phase of treatment. The long-term plan for Hirschsprung's disease involves another surgery, typically when the child is a bit older and stronger, to remove the affected segment of the intestine and reconnect the healthy parts. This procedure, known as a pull-through surgery, would eventually eliminate the need for the colostomy.

For now, the patient was ready for discharge from the NICU. The family was given detailed instructions on colostomy care, signs of complications to watch for, and the importance of regular follow-up visits. The transition from the NICU to home is always a critical period, but we ensured that the family was well-prepared and had access to all necessary resources and support.

# CHAPTER TWENTY

## NEONATAL HERPES

THE PATIENT WAS ADMITTED to the Neonatal Intensive Care Unit (NICU) within the first 48 hours of life with symptoms indicative of a serious infection. Born full-term to a mother with no significant prenatal history, the initial Apgar scores were 8 and 9 at one and five minutes, respectively. However, within the first 24 hours, the patient began to exhibit signs of systemic illness, including irritability, poor feeding, lethargy, and episodes of apnea. A physical examination revealed vesicular lesions on the scalp and trunk, a telltale sign of neonatal herpes simplex virus (HSV) infection.

Given the clinical presentation and the critical nature of neonatal HSV infection, an immediate diagnostic workup was initiated. Blood, cerebrospinal fluid (CSF), and swab samples from the lesions were collected for HSV PCR testing and culture. A complete blood count (CBC) revealed leukopenia with a marked left shift, and the patient's C-reactive protein (CRP) levels were elevated, indicating an inflammatory response.

The results of the diagnostic tests confirmed the presence of HSV-2 DNA in both the blood and CSF, establishing the diagnosis of disseminated neonatal herpes simplex infection with central nervous system (CNS) involvement. This form of HSV infection is associated with significant morbidity and mortality, thus warranting immediate and aggressive treatment.

The treatment plan for the patient was multifaceted, involving antiviral therapy, supportive care, and monitoring for potential complications. Intravenous (IV) acyclovir was initiated at a dose of 60 mg/kg/day, divided into three doses, to be administered over a period of 21 days. This dosage was based on the established protocol for treating neonatal HSV infections, aiming to maximize the drug's efficacy while minimizing potential toxicity.

In addition to the antiviral therapy, the patient required comprehensive supportive care. Due to poor feeding and the risk of dehydration, total parenteral nutrition (TPN) was started to ensure adequate caloric and fluid intake. An umbilical venous catheter was placed for the administration of TPN and other medications.

The patient also exhibited respiratory distress, likely secondary to CNS involvement and systemic inflammation. To manage this, a high-flow nasal cannula (HFNC) was used to deliver supplemental oxygen and support respiratory function. Continuous monitoring of oxygen saturation, heart rate, and respiratory rate was essential to promptly address any episodes of apnea or desaturation.

Seizures are a common complication in neonatal HSV infections with CNS involvement. Prophylactic anticonvulsant therapy was initiated with phenobarbital, starting with a loading dose of 20 mg/kg IV, followed by a maintenance dose of 5 mg/kg/day. Continuous electroencephalogram (EEG) monitoring was implemented to detect and manage any subclinical seizures.

To address the risk of secondary bacterial infections, broad-spectrum antibiotics were administered empirically until bacterial cultures from the blood and CSF returned negative. The chosen antibiotics included ampicillin and gentamicin, dosed according to neonatal guidelines, to cover a wide range of potential pathogens.

Throughout the treatment period, the patient's clinical status was closely monitored. Daily assessments included physical examinations, repeat blood work, and imaging studies. Cranial ultrasounds were performed to evaluate for any signs of intracranial complications such as hemorrhage or hydrocephalus, both of which can occur in severe HSV infections.

Despite the aggressive treatment and supportive care, the patient's condition remained critical. The vesicular lesions continued to spread, and the patient exhibited persistent signs of systemic illness. Repeat HSV PCR testing showed a decrease in viral load, but the clinical improvement was minimal.

On the 15th day of hospitalization, the patient developed signs of multi-organ dysfunction, including worsening respiratory distress, hypotension, and oliguria. Dopamine and dobutamine infusions were started to support cardiac function and maintain adequate blood pressure. The patient was also placed on a mechanical ventilator due to progressive respiratory failure.

Laboratory tests revealed a worsening metabolic acidosis and rising liver enzymes, indicative of hepatic involvement, a known complication of disseminated HSV infection. A decision was made to perform a liver ultrasound, which showed signs of hepatic necrosis.

The patient's condition continued to deteriorate despite all efforts. On the 18th day, the patient developed severe disseminated intravascular coagulation

(DIC), characterized by bleeding from multiple sites, including the catheter insertion points and the gastrointestinal tract. Fresh frozen plasma and platelet transfusions were administered to manage the coagulopathy.

Unfortunately, on the 20th day of life, the patient went into cardiac arrest. Despite resuscitation efforts, including chest compressions, epinephrine administration, and advanced cardiac life support protocols, the patient could not be revived and was pronounced dead.

Despite timely diagnosis and aggressive treatment, the prognosis for such cases remains poor, highlighting the need for early detection and preventive measures in at-risk populations.

Continue with
Stories From the NICU: Volume 4

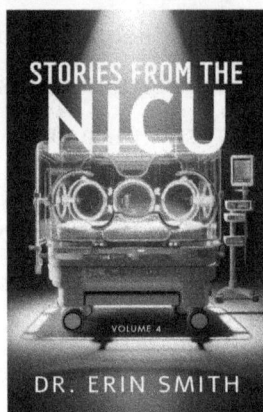

Dr. Erin Smith is a distinguished physician and author, originally hailing from the warm, vibrant landscapes of Alabama. With a career spanning over two decades, she has carved a niche for herself in the medical field, earning respect and admiration from colleagues and patients alike. Dr. Smith's journey in medicine has been marked by her unwavering dedication, sharp intellect, and a heartfelt passion for making a difference in the lives of others.

After completing her medical training in Alabama, Dr. Smith decided to spread her wings and bring her Southern charm and expertise to new horizons. She eventually settled outside of Salt Lake City, where she has continued to thrive both professionally and personally.

In addition to her demanding career, Dr. Smith is a devoted wife and the proud mother of two energetic sons. Balancing her professional responsibilities with her role as a mother has been a rewarding challenge, and she credits her family for providing her with the strength and support to excel in every facet of her life.

Dr. Smith's unique ability to connect with her patients, combined with her flair for storytelling, led her to compile and share her and her colleagues experiences in both, *Crazy Medical Stories* and *Stories From the NICU*.

With her roots firmly planted in her Alabama heritage, and her branches extending to nurture her family and career in Utah, Dr. Erin Smith stands as a remarkable figure in medicine—a doctor with a heart as big as her intellect, and stories as captivating as her journey.

ALSO BY FREE REIGN PUBLISHING

www.ingramcontent.com/pod-product-compliance
Lightning Source LLC
Chambersburg PA
CBHW022041190326
41520CB00008B/673